EXCHANGES
FOR ALL
OCCASIONS

Your Guide to
Choosing Healthy Foods
Anytime Anywhere

Marion J. Franz, MS, RD, CDE

IDC Publishing
Minneapolis

This book presents general guidelines for developing a personal meal plan. If you have a health condition that requires a therapeutic meal plan, you should consult your health care provider.

IDC Publishing
3800 Park Nicollet Boulevard
Minneapolis, Minnesota 55416-2699
(612) 993-3393
www.idcpublishing.com

Library of Congress Cataloging-in-Publication Data
Franz, Marion J.
    Exchanges for all occasions : your guide to choosing healthy foods anytime, anywhere / Marion J. Franz. — 4th ed.
    Third ed., rev. and expanded published with subtitle: How to use the exchange system for healthy and creative food choices.
    Includes index.
    ISBN 1-885115-35-0
1. Diabetes—Diet therapy. 2. Diabetes—Nutritional aspects. 3. Food exchange lists. I. Title.
RC662.F734 1997
616.4'620654—dc21   97-12307
                                                                CIP

Editorial Director/Publisher: Karol Carstensen
Assistant Editor: Sara Frueh
Production Manager: Gail Devery
Cover and Text Design: MacLean & Tuminelly

Printed in the United States of America

Distributed to bookstores by Chronimed Publishing, Minneapolis, Minnesota

Table of Contents

Foreword 5

**PART ONE   Exchanges, Meal Planning,
             and Nutrition** 7
Chapter 1   Good Nutrition, Good Health 9
Chapter 2   Meal Planning Made Easy 15
Chapter 3   Maintaining a Reasonable Weight 25
Chapter 4   Cutting Back on Fat 31
Chapter 5   Sugar, Salt, and Fiber 41

**PART TWO   Using Exchanges in
             Everyday Life** 51
Chapter 6   Using Food Labels 53
Chapter 7   Cooking With Exchanges 67
Chapter 8   Dining Out With Exchanges 77
Chapter 9   Travel and Meal Planning 89

PART THREE Carbohydrate Exchange Lists 97
Chapter 10   Starch List 99
Chapter 11   Fruit and Vegetable Lists 113
Chapter 12   Milk List 121
Chapter 13   Other Carbohydrates List 125

**PART FOUR   Meat, Fat, and Other
             Exchange Lists** 131
Chapter 14   Meat and Meat Substitutes List 133
Chapter 15   Fat List 147
Chapter 16   Free Foods List 151
Chapter 17   Combination Foods List 155

PART FIVE   Ethnic Exchanges **161**

Chapter 18   Vegetarian Exchanges 163
Chapter 19   Asian Food Exchanges 175
Chapter 20   Exchanges Mexican Style 189
Chapter 21   Exchanges Italiano....................... 201
Chapter 22   Spicy Indian Exchanges 209
Chapter 23   Exchanges for Jewish Cookery 219

PART SIX   Exchanges on the Go.............. 227

Chapter 24   Exchanges for the Fast Food
              Phenomenon 229
Chapter 25   Exchanges for Convenience Foods 243
Chapter 26   Exchanges for Smart Snacking............. 249
Chapter 27   Exchanges for Camping................... 261

APPENDICES.............................. 269

Appendix 1   Resources 271
Appendix 2   More on Fat Replacers................... 275
Appendix 3   Common Sugars and Sweeteners.......... 279
Appendix 4   Calculating Exchanges From
              Food Labels 283
Appendix 5   Foreign Language Phrases for
              People With Diabetes................... 287
Appendix 6   Glossary of Food Terms................. 289

References................................ 311

Index 313

Foreword

Change—it's the one thing that is always certain. Changes happen in medical care, politics, sports, and even families. Changes also happen to books and *Exchanges for All Occasions* is no exception. This is the fourth edition, and I hope that with each edition the book has become more useful for readers.

This edition of *Exchanges for All Occasions* is based on the 1995 Exchange Lists for Meal Planning of the American Diabetes Association and The American Dietetic Association and incorporates carbohydrate counting along with the exchange system. For those readers to whom carbohydrate counting is a new idea, it is a system of meal planning used more and more frequently by people with diabetes. It simply means that all foods containing primarily carbohydrate—starches, fruits, milk, sweets, and vegetables—are carbohydrate choices; it doesn't mean you ignore calories, protein, and fat. A new column showing carbohydrate choices appears in this edition along with a column showing exchange values.

The order of the book has changed as well. The basics of healthy nutrition and food are covered in Part One. Part Two deals with the practicalities of making food selections every day—food purchasing and preparation, eating out, and travel. Parts Three and Four are the heart of the book; they contain the basic lists of food choices with their exchange and carbohydrate choice values.

Vegetarian and ethnic foods add variety and spice to meal planning. Information and exchange values for these interesting foods are in Part Five, including a new chapter on Indian foods. And finally Part Six deals with an ever-growing facet of food selection—fast foods, convenience foods, and snack foods.

Over the years two things have not changed. One is the growing appreciation for the importance of good nutrition in the prevention and management of many chronic health problems. Through good nutrition and physical activity we can all hear "the sound of cheering from within," which gives us energy and enthusiasm for all the good things life has to offer!

The second thing that has not changed is my gratitude to all who continue to make this book possible. A very special thanks my colleagues—the supportive and highly skilled dietitians at the International Diabetes Center—Betty Bajwa (especially for her help with the chapter on Indian foods), Barbara Barry, Gay Castle, Nancy Cooper, Jill Flader, Joy Jocelyn, Arlene Monk, Diane Reader, and Angie Sharp, as well as several nutrition students who helped gather information for the book. Also, the feedback and appreciation from dietitians and other health educators around the United States (and the world) has been truly appreciated. It is wonderful to know that others have found the book helpful to themselves as professionals as well as to the public they serve.

No book could be written without the assistance of a publishing staff. A large vote of thanks to Karol Carstensen, Director of IDC Publishing, Gail Devery, and Sara Frueh. Their ideas, editing suggestions, and support were invaluable. Not to be forgotten are the rest of the entire International Diabetes Center staff—from Richard M. Bergenstal, M.D., Executive Director, to Kay Martin, Administrative Assistant—for their continued support and encouragement. All forty-eight of you continue to be grand!

Marion J. Franz, MS, RD, CDE

PART ONE

Exchanges, Meal Planning, and Nutrition

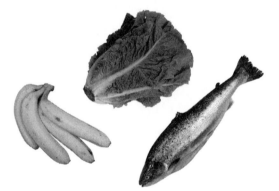

CHAPTER 1

Good Nutrition, Good Health

Good nutrition and good health begin with making healthy food choices. Regular physical activity is equally important to good health and contributes to the success of any healthy eating plan. Eating a balanced, healthy diet and staying physically active help you look and feel your best.

While the importance of physical activity to your health and well being can't be stressed enough, this book is about food. Scientists have made great strides in understanding the role of food and nutrition in health and disease, and we now know that healthy food choices not only improve health but can actually help prevent some health problems. Making healthy food choices, along with living an active lifestyle, can reduce your risk of obesity, heart disease, diabetes, high blood pressure, and some forms of cancer.

In spite of all that's known about the importance of healthy eating, changing eating habits isn't easy for most people. Adopting healthy eating habits is a long-term proposition, and success can easily be thwarted by a short-term approach. That's the problem with most "diets." They may work, but many are so restrictive or impractical that it's impossible to stay on them. As soon as you revert to your old eating habits, you revert to your old health risks as well.

To make permanent changes in your eating habits, you need to find ways to fit the foods you enjoy into your everyday life. If you love ice cream, for instance, it usually doesn't work to swear off it forever. Eating smaller amounts less often, or switching to light ice cream or frozen yogurt would be more practical, and even a small change toward healthier eating is better than no change. The key is to make reasonable changes that you can stick to over the long run. You also need tools that can help you make good food choices in any situation, whether you're enjoying a home-cooked meal, stopping by a fast food restaurant, or celebrating at a New Year's Eve party.

The goal is to provide you with the information and tools that can help you design a personal plan of eating based on your food preferences, your lifestyle, your nutrition needs, and your health goals. Next, a comprehensive listing of a variety of foods along with the information you need to include them in your meals in a healthy way is provided. These are the exchange lists.

Meal Planning

A meal plan is a personalized guide to what you need to eat each day to meet your nutrition and health goals. For instance, if weight loss is your goal but you are a real "cookie monster," a personal meal plan in conjunction with wise food choices will help you satisfy your cookie craving and still lose weight. It can be done!

Weight loss or control is just one reason to have and follow a meal plan. People with high blood cholesterol levels or heart problems also can benefit from a meal plan that helps them control their fat intake. Diets high in saturated fat contribute to the development of artherosclerosis and heart disease which can lead to heart attack. And people who have diabetes need a meal plan that tells them how much carbohydrate and fat they need to eat at meals and snacks in order to control their blood glucose (sugar) and blood cholesterol levels. Carbohydrate foods make blood glucose levels rise more than other foods, yet they are essential to a healthy diet. Also, people with diabetes are at risk for developing heart disease. A meal plan helps them include carbohydrate foods in their diets, reduce fat, and maintain healthy blood glucose levels.

If you already have a meal plan, the lists and information in this book will help you follow it in almost any setting or situation you are likely to be. If you have a particular health condition, like diabetes, and don't have a meal plan, you need to have one developed for you. Usually this is done by a registered dietitian. The appendix lists resources that can help you find a dietitian in your area, or you can ask your health care provider to refer you to one.

Even if you don't have a health condition that requires a meal plan, you can benefit by following a plan of healthy eating. Besides enhancing good health, it is widely believed that adopting and following a healthy meal plan can help prevent or delay many health problems. If you want to eat more healthfully, and you don't need a meal plan for medical reasons, you can follow the steps in chapter 2 to design a plan for yourself.

Food Exchanges

Most meal plans are developed using the exchange system. The exchange system was established in the 1950s and has been revised several times as more has been learned about nutrition and how the body uses food. The American Diabetes Association and the American Dietetic Association adopted the system and developed the exchange lists. The lists help make meal planning easier for people wanting to control calories and fat, and for people with diabetes or other chronic diseases. The lists were most recently revised in 1995.

The exchange lists group foods based on nutritional content. The lists fall into three main groups: carbohydrate, meat and meat substitutes, and fat. Carbohydrate foods (starch, fruit, milk, other carbohydrates, and vegetables) provide energy. Meat and meat substitutes provide energy along with protein for growth, body repair, and body maintenance. Fats provide energy and carry the fat-soluble vitamins A, D, E and K. Together foods from these groups give us all the nutrients we need to live, grow, and stay healthy.

The Exchange Lists

Carbohydrate Lists
- Starch List
- Fruit List
- Milk List
- Other Carbohydrates List
- Vegetable List

Meat and Meat Substitutes List

Fat List

Free Foods List

Combination Foods List

Of course not all the foods we eat fit neatly into the three main groups. Lasagna, for instance, is made from pasta (starch), beef (meat), cheese (meat substitute), and tomato sauce (vegetable). The Combination Foods List accommodates such foods by giving serving sizes and the exchange values for each. The Free Foods List includes low-calorie, low-fat, low-sugar foods that can be used to round out your meals without worry.

Each list gives food choices and the amount of each food that equals one exchange, or one serving. Each serving from a list is a measured amount of food that has approximately the same carbohydrate, protein, fat, and caloric content as other foods on the same list. Any food on a list can be "exchanged," or traded, for any other food on the same list *in the amounts given*, because each serving provides the same nutritional value and the same number of calories.

Let's look at an example. Oatmeal and wheat bread are both on the Starch List. One serving of oatmeal is given as one-half cup, and one serving of wheat bread is one slice. Each of these servings is equal to one starch exchange. Therefore, if your meal plan included two starch exchanges for breakfast, you could choose to have one slice of wheat bread and one-half cup of oatmeal. Or you might choose to have two slices of wheat bread instead, and you would still be getting two starch exchanges. Similarly, you might choose to have one cup of oatmeal (two starch exchanges). This mix-and-match feature makes it easy to select from a wide variety of foods, giving you many choices to spice up your daily fare.

The lists in this book expand on the original exchange list idea by including more food choices in each of the basic exchange lists and by including exchange lists for different types of foods. The additional lists include more of the kinds of foods that are readily available today such as Indian foods, Mexican foods, Oriental foods, convenience foods and almost anything else you eat or want to eat. And you'll learn how to include the foods you like in your daily meal planning while meeting your nutrition and health goals.

Understanding Nutrition

When it comes to nutrition, it seems we're bombarded with constantly changing information. New fad diets appear with astonishing regularity, and while we would all like to believe that eating only grapefruit for a week or substituting a meal with a nutrient-rich drink once a day will result in a long, healthy and thin life, it just isn't so. Nor will a vitamin, mineral, or herbal supplement provide us with youth and health forever. Though the physical effects of these fad diets and supplements are not usually harmful, we can become increasingly discouraged as our hopes are lifted and dashed over and over by their unfulfilled promises. The most harmful result is that we give up all together.

With all the information and misinformation flying around, it's sometimes difficult to understand what good nutrition *is*. One of the simplest and most useful tools for understanding healthy eating is the Food Guide Pyramid. You may have seen the pyramid on food labels or in your doctor's office.

Created by the United States Department of Agriculture (USDA), the Food Guide Pyramid organizes food into six groups, graphically illustrating current nutrition guidelines. All of the food groups are essential for well-balanced, good nutrition, but as the pyramid shows, "well-balanced" doesn't mean eating equal amounts from all of the groups.

The pyramid ranks the major food groups by the role each should play in your total diet. Grains and starchy vegetables are at the base of the pyramid and are the foundation of good nutrition. Fruits and vegetables make up the next level and also are very important. Foods from these first two levels of the pyramid are emphasized in a healthy diet.

Milk and meat products are on the third level of the pyramid. They provide important nutrients, but also can contain fat. It's important to choose foods from these groups wisely, such as choosing low-fat or nonfat dairy products and lean meats. Meat is a special concern because the fat in it is easy to forget and yet can be quite substantial. Also, most of us probably eat more meat than is necessary for good nutrition and good health.

Fat and sweets (which often contain a lot of fat) are squeezed into the tip of the pyramid. Fat is necessary in the diet but, as the pyramid suggests, caution is required. A high-fat diet can contribute to weight gain as well as to the development of a host of chronic health conditions such as atherosclerosis and diabetes.

Do the pyramid food groups remind you of the exchange lists? If so, then you are well on your way to understanding how the lists can help you put the principles of the pyramid—the principles of good nutrition—into practice.

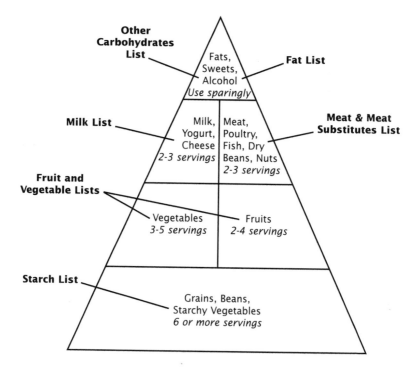

Food Guide Pyramid and Related Exchange Lists

Adapted from *Food Guide Pyramid*, © 1994,
U.S. Department of Agriculture

CHAPTER 2

Meal Planning Made Easy

A meal plan is like your own personal food pyramid—it tells you how many servings from each food group you need to eat each day for good nutrition and good health. But it goes one step further. A meal plan maps out for you how to allot your food group servings among the meals and snacks you normally eat over the course of a day. It tells you the servings from each of the food groups you need to eat at meals and snacks to meet your nutrition and health needs.

No one food or food group contains all the nutrients you need for good health, so it is important to eat a variety of foods each day. There are six nutrients in food, and each has a special role in our bodies. The nutrients are carbohydrate, protein, fat, vitamins, minerals, and water. The first three—carbohydrate, protein, and fat—provide the calories that give our bodies energy and are the primary focus in meal planning. The last three nutrients—vitamins, minerals, and water—help regulate our body processes and do not provide any calories. The daily requirements for vitamins and minerals are usually satisfied by a balanced diet built around appropriate amounts of carbohydrate, protein, and fat.

The foods we eat are often described by the nutrients they contain. For instance pasta is a carbohydrate food, and meat is a protein and fat food. Carbohydrate and protein each provide four calories per gram, and fat provides nine calories per gram. Alcohol also has calories. It provides seven calories per gram. (A gram is about the weight of a paper clip, and there are thirty grams in one ounce.)

Carbohydrate Foods

Carbohydrate foods are found on the following exchange lists: Starch List, Fruit List, Milk List, Vegetable List, and Other Carbohydrates List. Carbohydrate is the body's first choice for energy. The number of servings of carbohydrate foods that you need depends on your total daily calorie needs. Approximately half of your daily calories should be from carbohydrate foods.

There are three different types of carbohydrate: starch, sugar, and fiber. Chemically, all carbohydrates are actually made from different types of sugar. Starches are often called complex carbohydrates, and sugars are often called simple carbohydrates. Fiber is a carbohydrate that the body cannot break down or digest.

Starch is present in grains, pasta, cereal, and starchy vegetables like potatoes and winter squash. Sugar occurs naturally in milk, fruit, and vegetables. Table sugar and foods with added sugar such as soft drinks and sweets also are carbohydrate sources, but you should use them in moderation. They are "empty calories" that provide no important nutrients. Fiber is found in whole-grain breads and cereals, fruits, vegetables, and dried peas, beans, and lentils. Foods containing fiber provide bulk to the diet and usually are good sources of vitamins and minerals as well, so they are good food choices. The following table lists carbohydrate foods that are good sources of fiber.

Food	Serving Size	Grams of Fiber (average)
Starch		
Breads: whole wheat, whole grain, or crackers	1 slice or 1 oz	2
Cereals: dry or cooked	varies	3
Bran cereals	⅓–½ cup	8
Starchy vegetables: potatoes, brown rice, green peas	½ cup	3
Legumes: peas, beans, lentils	⅓ cup	4–5
Grains: kasha, couscous, bulgur, wild rice	½ cup	2
Fruit		
Fresh, frozen, or canned	½ cup	2
Fresh	1 small	2
Vegetable		
Cooked, canned, or frozen	½–¾ cup	2
Raw	1–2 cups	3

Protein Foods

Foods on the Meat and Meat Substitutes List are sources of protein. Milk and milk products, besides supplying carbohydrate, also are sources of protein. Protein from food is digested and enters the bloodstream as amino acids. Amino acids are used to form new tissue or to repair damaged tissue. Most Americans get two to three times as much protein as they actually need. Two to three servings of a protein source such as meat, fish, poultry, cheese, milk, or eggs fill the daily protein requirement for most people. Protein foods often contain a lot of fat, so choose lean meats and low-fat or non-fat dairy foods.

Fat Foods

Foods that are primarily fat are on the Fat List; these include butter, margarine, oils, and salad dressings. Meat, many dairy foods, many snack and prepared foods, and desserts also contain large amounts of fat. The fat in food supplies a concentrated form of energy that is needed for proper body function. Though some fat in our diets is necessary to perform these functions, most of us eat too much. You should get no more than thirty percent of your daily calories from fat.

There are three main types of fat: saturated, polyunsaturated, and monounsaturated. Usually, all are present in foods that contain fat. Monounsaturated or polyunsaturated fats are preferable to saturated fats because saturated fats can raise your blood cholesterol levels and increase your risk for heart problems. How do you tell the difference? In general, unsaturated fats are liquid at room temperature, while saturated fats are solid or semi-solid at room temperature.

Calories

In addition to eating the foods that give you the nutrients you need, it is important to eat enough food each day to meet your caloric requirements. Your meal plan is based on your daily calorie needs. Normal weight adults need to consume enough calories to maintain their weight. Children and adolescents usually require larger numbers of calories than adults to provide for their energy and growth. They *do not* need a meal plan that is restricted in calories, nor do they need excessive calories in relation to their energy needs.

Nutrient	Function	Some Food Sources
Carbohydrate	The body's first choice for energy or fuel. Carbohydrates affect blood glucose levels the most, which is relevant for people who have diabetes.	
	Sugars (natural and added) are an energy source. They also are carbohydrate in its simplest form.	*Natural:* Fruits, vegetables, milk; *Added:* Table sugar, honey, soft drinks, syrup, candies, pies, cakes, cookies, jams, and jellies
	Starches are made up of many sugars that are linked together in long chains.	Breads, cereals, pastas, grains, rice, and starchy vegetables such as potatoes, corn, peas, lima beans, and squash
	Fiber is the "structure" in some foods. It is not digested by the body, and it helps the body remove waste.	Whole-grain breads and cereals, fruits, vegetables, and legumes (dried beans, peas, and lentils)
Protein	Essential for forming new tissue, repairing damaged tissue, and maintaining muscle, skin, and blood health. Some also can be changed into glucose for energy.	Meat, fish, poultry, cheese, eggs, milk, dried beans, peas and lentils, nuts, and seeds
Fat 10% or less of daily intake should be from saturated fats	A concentrated energy source that provides essential fatty acids for normal body function. Fat also is one of the body's main sources of energy.	
	Polyunsaturated and Monounsaturated Fats are liquid at room temperature and can help lower blood cholesterol levels.	Most vegetable oils: olive, canola, peanut, corn, cottonseed, safflower, soybean, sunflower; olives, peanuts, walnuts
	Saturated Fats are solid at room temperature and raise blood cholesterol levels.	Butter, cheese, meats, lard, palm oil, coconut oil, cocoa butter, solid vegetable shortenings

Some people, especially those with weight or health problems, may need a meal plan that helps them lose weight. However, no meal plan should be so restrictive in calories that it is impossible to follow. Cutting just 500 calories from your daily intake can produce a consistent, gradual weight loss; a faster, more drastic weight loss, while initially exhilarating, can be difficult to maintain. Even a moderate weight loss of ten to twenty pounds can help improve health factors such as blood cholesterol, blood fats (triglycerides), blood pressure, and blood glucose.

The lowest calorie intake recommended for adult women is 1200 to 1400 calories a day; 1500 to 1800 calories is the daily minimum for adult men. If you need to lose weight and are unable to while on a minimum-calorie diet, you need to increase your caloric expenditure through exercise rather than eat less. Studies have shown that people who include regular physical activity as part of their weight control program are more successful at sticking to their program and keeping the weight off. Reaching and maintaining a healthy weight is discussed in more detail in chapter 3.

Three Steps to a Healthy Meal Plan

You can develop your own meal plan by following three simple steps.

Step 1. Determine your daily calorie needs by multiplying as follows.

Most men and very active women:
Current weight in pounds _____ x 15 = _____ calories

Inactive men and most women:
Current weight in pounds _____ x 13 = _____ calories

If you want to lose weight:
Current weight in pounds _____ x 10 = _____ calories

Step 2. Using your answer to Step 1 and the Daily Servings chart below, determine how many servings from each food group you need each day.

Daily Servings Based on Calorie Needs

	~1500	1600–1900	2000–2300	2400–2700
Carbohydrate (starch, fruit, milk, or other carbohydrate)	10–12	13–15	16–18	19–21
Vegetable	as desired	as desired	as desired	as desired
Meat	1½ (4–5 oz)	2 (6 oz)	2 (6 oz)	2½ (6–8 oz)
Fat	3–4	4–5	4–5	5–6

Step 3. Use the number of servings from Step 2 to fill out your meal plan on page 21. A 1500-calorie meal plan is shown as an example. The example lists the total number of carbohydrate choices and then divides these choices into starch, fruit, and milk exchanges to show a well-balanced diet.

Be sure to allot your servings according to the meals and snacks you normally eat. If you don't usually eat a snack in the morning, you don't need to include one in your plan. However, if you do eat snacks, be sure to plan for them so that you don't eat "extra" at those times.

Most nutrition and health experts believe that snacks, along with regular small meals, help to keep energy levels up throughout the day and to control appetite. This decreases the likelihood of overeating at meals and can help with weight loss and control as well as blood glucose and blood cholesterol control. Carbohydrate foods from the starch, fruit, or milk exchange lists are good choices for snacks because carbohydrate is the body's main source of energy.

Following a meal plan that distributes carbohydrate foods throughout the day helps keep your body fueled and functioning well. This is especially important if you have diabetes. Blood glucose control is best achieved by consistently feeding your body carbohydrate in small amounts throughout the day. This is discussed further later in this chapter. If you do have diabetes or another health problem, be sure to discuss your nutrition needs with your health care provider.

Sample 1500-Calorie Meal Plan

	Breakfast	Snack	Lunch	Snack	Dinner	Snack	Total
Carbohydrate	4	0–1	3	1	3	0–1	12
Starch	2	0–1	2		3	0–1	8
Fruit	1			1			2
Milk	1		1				2
Vegetable			1		2		2–3
Meat	0–1		1 (1–2 oz)		1 (3–4 oz)		2 (4–5 oz)
Fat	1		1–2		1–2		3–4

My Meal Plan

	Breakfast	Snack	Lunch	Snack	Dinner	Snack	Total
Carbohydrate							
Starch							
Fruit							
Milk							
Vegetable							
Meat							
Fat							

Your meal plan is like a puzzle; all you need to do now is use the exchange lists in this book to choose the foods you like and fit them into your plan. Remember that it's also important to choose a wide variety of foods for a balanced diet and for good health. And if you decide to eat a food from the Other Carbohydrates List, be sure to count it in your meal plan by substituting it for a starch, a fruit, or a milk choice.

Almost any food can be included in your meal plan if you are guided by one simple principle: moderation. Next to making healthy food choices, controlling portion sizes is the most important part of healthy eating. The exchange lists help you by giving the portion size that is equal to one serving of a food. You might want to use measuring cups and a small food scale at first to get used to the appropriate serving sizes of different foods. Get to know what one-half cup of your favorite cereal looks like in your bowl and how much of your plate is taken up by three ounces of fish. After awhile you will be able to accurately "eyeball" your servings. But beware, serving sizes of most desserts and fat-filled snacks are quite small. It will help if you can learn to get satisfaction from the taste of these foods in small amounts, and to eat them only occasionally, rather than trying to "fill up" on them on a regular basis.

Carbohydrate Counting and Diabetes

Carbohydrate counting is a meal planning method used in diabetes. It simply means that food choices made from any of the carbohydrate exchange lists will count as carbohydrates in the meal plan. This allows more flexibility in meal planning than does an exchange meal plan in which specific guidelines for starch, fruit, and milk exchanges are given. Carbohydrate counting is based on the fact that any of these choices will have the same effect on blood glucose levels.

The goals of meal planning in diabetes are to keep blood sugar (glucose) levels in control (as near normal as possible) and to keep blood fats (cholesterol and triglycerides) in an ideal range. Counting carbohydrates helps people with diabetes control blood glucose levels, but while it is a simple and effective meal planning tool, the danger is that fat content and calories may be ignored. It is still important for people with diabetes to watch their meat and fat intake, just as it is for everybody.

One carbohydrate choice has fifteen grams of carbohydrate and is equal to one starch, one fruit, one milk, or one other carbohydrate exchange. Most adults need three to four carbohydrate choices at meals and one to two at snacks. Children and teenagers will need more.

People who inject insulin need a meal plan that provides a consistent amount of carbohydrate at the same times each day. By eating consistently and by monitoring blood glucose levels, insulin therapy can be appropriately designed and integrated with food habits to achieve the best blood glucose control possible. It also is possible to learn how to adjust the amount of carbohydrate foods you eat or the insulin doses you take to help blood glucose control.

Meal planning is a little different for people with type II diabetes treated with nutrition therapy alone or with nutrition therapy and oral medications. In this case, the amount of food and fat eaten needs to be decreased, and carbohydrate intake needs to be spread throughout the day. Success is enhanced by making good food choices, learning new eating behaviors, and increasing physical activity. Also, losing even a small amount of weight (ten to twenty pounds) can improve blood glucose levels and reduce the need for medications.

Both the exchange system and carbohydrate counting can be effectively used by people with diabetes. We have included both exchanges and carbohydrate choices in the lists in this book.

If you have diabetes and don't have a meal plan, a registered dietitian can help you develop one. To locate a registered dietitian in your area, ask your health care provider, call your local hospital or public health department, or call The American Dietetic Association's Nutrition Hotline at 1-800-366-1655.

Keys to Success

In today's busy world, it's hard enough for most of us just to get a meal on the table let alone worry about a meal plan. Following a meal plan on a daily basis *can* be difficult. That's why it's important to do everything you can to create built-in support for your meal planning efforts. While everyone has their own way of approaching it, the following have proven to be effective aids to long-term success.

- Recognize your meal plan as a tool for good health. It is not a set menu or diet. Rather, it is a guide that will allow you to take charge of your eating habits and your health.

- Seek support from family and friends. Having family members eat the same healthy foods that you do and join you in regular physical activity, such as walking, bike riding, and swimming can help reinforce your meal planning efforts over time.

- Focus on personal motivation. People who shift their thinking from "I am doing this because my family wants me to or because my doctor told me to" to "I am doing this for myself and to be in charge of my life" tend to follow their meal plans better than those who do not.

- Focus on positive changes in health risks. For example, improved self-esteem, higher energy levels, improved blood glucose or cholesterol levels, and reduced blood pressure are more important than what the scale says.

- Get and stay physically active. Physical activity is the strongest predictor of long-term adherence to healthy meal planning.

In Summary

As you think about incorporating your meal plan and healthy eating into your life, remember: good food, good health, good taste. Too often we equate a diet rich in fat, cholesterol, sugar, calories, and salt with good-tasting food. However, this is not necessarily true. Healthy food can and does taste good.

CHAPTER 3

Maintaining a Reasonable Weight

If you consume more food than your body needs, the calories are stored as energy reserves, or fat. This is true even when you eat healthy, low-fat foods because *any* extra calories can be stored as fat. Fat is a very efficient means of storage, and the body has an almost limitless capacity to accumulate fatty tissue. Unfortunately, our talent for storing energy as fat is not much of a "plus." Excess weight contributes to a number of chronic diseases such as heart disease, arthritis, breathing problems, and diabetes. In short, carrying around extra weight is a strain on your body and your health.

The location of body fat matters as well. You may have heard there's an advantage to being a "pear" rather than an "apple." This means that it's better to carry excess weight in the hips and thighs (pear) than to carry it in the abdomen or stomach (apple). Extra fat in the stomach area is linked to diabetes and early heart disease.

This chapter will help you learn if you need to lose weight, how much to lose, and how best to do it. The bottom line is that losing small amounts of weight and keeping it off can have major health benefits.

Finding Your Healthy Weight

Just as we accept that some people are shorter or taller than average, we also need to accept the fact that some people will weigh more or less than average. Healthy weight ranges for adult men and women of all ages are shown in the figure below. The higher rates in your healthy weight range apply to people who are more muscular or have large bones. The further you are above the healthy weight range for your height, the higher your weight-related health risk. Weights below your range are not necessarily better either, though being slightly underweight may be normal for some people. Unintentional weight loss may signal a health problem.

Are You Overweight?

Height*

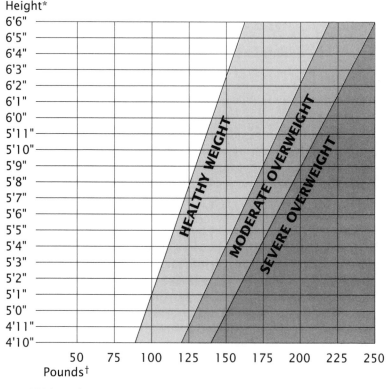

* Without shoes.

† Without clothes. The higher weights apply to people with more muscle and bone, such as many men.

Source: *Dietary Guidelines for Americans*, fourth edition, 1995; U.S. Department of Agriculture and U.S. Department of Health and Human Services

What determines which area of the weight spectrum we wind up in? Genetics is one major factor. Studies have shown that the adult weights of identical twins separated at birth and raised in different environments are identical. Also, adults who were adopted as children are closer in weight to their biological parents than to their adopted parents. If you have a family history of obesity, you may have to work harder at maintaining a reasonable weight, and you may have to set a weight goal that is slightly higher than what is typically recommended for your height, age, and gender. Striving for a pencil-slim figure may simply be unrealistic.

An "ideal" body weight is often elusive, and the quest is often frustrating. It is more beneficial to concentrate on making healthy food choices and on participating in regular, moderate physical activity. This will improve your weight, your overall health, and your self-esteem.

Do You Need to Lose Weight?

To answer this question, you need to consider your healthy weight range from the chart on page 26, your family history, and your current eating and activity habits. If your weight is in the healthy range in the chart and you have gained less than ten pounds since you reached your adult height, you don't need to lose weight. Your goal is to prevent weight gain, especially as you age. If you are eating healthfully and getting regular physical activity and you are in the moderate overweight range in the chart, you may need to accept that this weight is normal and healthy for you. However, if you are in the severe overweight range and inactive, you will undoubtedly benefit from making some lifestyle changes that can help you lose weight. This is especially important if you have a weight-related medical problem or a family history of such problems.

The good news is that weight loss doesn't need to be dramatic to improve your health or decrease health risks. Losing even a small amount of weight can lead to big health gains. One study, for example, found that participants who lost ten percent of their body weight increased their "good" (HDL) cholesterol level. In another study, people who lost fifteen percent of their body weight also reduced their blood pressure by ten percent. A third study found that people with diabetes who lost just twenty pounds decreased their blood glucose levels and their need for medication. People at risk for diabetes and some other chronic diseases also can help reduce their chances of ever getting the disease by controlling their weight.

Setting Reasonable Goals

To lose weight, you must burn more calories than you consume. It's a simple concept, but if you've tried to lose weight before you know it's hard to achieve. One of the keys to success is making reasonable changes in your eating habits that you think you can stick to permanently. Perhaps you already have a meal plan that will help you lose weight. If not, chapter 2 will help you determine how many calories you need to eat each day in order to lose weight, and it will help you build a meal plan based on those calories.

It's a common misconception that if you don't eat fat, you will lose weight. This misconception has contributed to an enormous increase in the manufacture and consumption of fat-free foods. But the only way to lose weight is to eat fewer calories than you need to maintain your current weight. It is even possible to lose weight eating nothing but fat, if the total calories are at a level that promotes weight loss. (Obviously this is not recommended.) One good reason to watch fat is that, gram for gram, fat has more calories that carbohydrate or protein. So if you cut back on fat and refrain from getting those calories from some other source (like fat-free foods), you can lose weight.

The goal of weight management is to lose small amounts of weight, then keep those pounds off for a lifetime. If you need to lose weight, decide on a weight goal that is reasonable for you to reach and to maintain over the long run. It's important to lose weight gradually, as you make changes in your eating and activity habits. Strive to lose from one-half to two pounds each week. As you lose weight, your body will become more efficient at using energy, and your rate of weight loss may decrease. If you hit a plateau, increased physical activity is the best way to continue losing weight and to avoid gaining it back.

Physical Activity

If you want to lose weight and keep it off, you also must be willing to commit to some form of regular physical activity. Ninety percent of all individuals who do well with weight maintenance and weight loss report becoming involved with an exercise program. Luckily, physical activity doesn't have to mean a high-intensity aerobics class or countless laps around a jogging track. Opportunities for physical activity are all around you—walking the dog, gardening, and housework all burn calories and help you stay healthy.

If you're currently inactive, start by walking around the block each day. After a week of sticking to this plan, increase it to walking around two blocks, and so on. Whatever activity you choose, build up gradually to a total of thirty minutes of light to moderate activity on most days of the week. If you can't do the thirty minutes at one time, you can spread them throughout the day. A ten-minute walk before breakfast, taking the stairs at work, and a short lunch-time stroll can add up to your daily dose of fitness.

Seek Support

Look for support in your weight loss efforts. Most people cannot do it themselves. Family or friends are important if you are to be successful. No matter how determined you are, if people close to you are not supportive of your lifestyle changes, they can easily sabotage your attempts. Here are a few suggestions to help you build support.

- Ask a friend or family member to go for a walk with you.
- Buy a piece of home exercise equipment that the whole family can use.
- Shop for healthy foods with your family.
- Ask your family to help you keep high-fat snacks out of the house.
- Ask a co-worker to walk with you during your lunch hour.
- Start a contest at work to see who climbs the most stairs in a week.

Professional assistance also may be helpful, as obesity can be a lifelong health problem. During the next five to ten years, new medications that can assist with maintaining weight loss will be entering the market. Ask your doctor about the new generation of non-addictive prescription medications.

CHAPTER 4

Cutting Back on Fat

Diets high in fat are associated with obesity and an increased risk for diseases such as diabetes, some types of cancer, gallbladder disease, and coronary heart disease. Saturated fats in particular can increase blood cholesterol levels, which contributes to heart and other diseases and can lead to heart attack. Heart disease and heart attacks are special concerns because they are so prevalent in our population. People with a family history of heart disease and people with diabetes are especially at risk for heart disease and heart attack.

Most heart attacks occur in people with blood cholesterol levels between 200 and 240. Approximately half of all adults have total cholesterol levels above 200. If your blood cholesterol is high, reducing it by just one percent will decrease your risk of coronary heart disease by two percent.

Cholesterol

Cholesterol is a fat-like, waxy substance. The body needs cholesterol to make hormones and to support and protect cells. The body makes the cholesterol it requires. In the diet, cholesterol comes from animal foods such as meat, poultry, egg yolks, and fat-containing dairy products. The effect of food cholesterol on blood cholesterol varies from person to person. Even foods that do not contain cholesterol can be high in total and saturated fat, which are bigger concerns.

Lipoproteins transport fats and cholesterol throughout the bloodstream to the cells where they are used or stored. There are several kinds of lipoproteins, but two are especially important in determining risk for coronary heart disease. *LDL-cholesterol* carries most of the cholesterol through the arteries in the body. When there is too much LDL-cholesterol in the bloodstream, it combines with other substances to form a plaque and narrows the blood vessels. When this happens, less blood reaches the heart and a heart attack can happen. *HDL-cholesterol* carries cholesterol away from the arteries and to the liver where the liver can dispose of it. HDL-cholesterol, also known as "good" cholesterol, protects against heart disease. You can improve your HDL-cholesterol level with a routine that includes regular physical activity.

In addition to high blood cholesterol levels, high triglyceride levels, especially in people with diabetes, also are a risk for heart disease. Triglycerides are food fats. Triglycerides also are the way fats are transported through the bloodstream and the way fat is stored in fat cells.

A diet low or moderate in saturated fats can help reduce blood cholesterol and triglyceride levels and lower your risk of heart disease. A low-fat diet overall can reduce your calorie intake and the risk of other diseases, like some cancers. The question is: Are you eating too much fat and, if you are, how can you cut back on fat and still eat foods that are tasty and that you enjoy?

How Much Fat Is Too Much

Health experts recommend consuming no more than thirty percent of total daily calories from fat and no more than ten percent from saturated fat. On average, Americans consume about thirty-four to thirty-eight percent of their total calories from fat and twelve percent from saturated fat. Statistics on fat consumption are similar in many other countries, such as Canada and many European nations, where food is abundant and where meat plays a central role in the diet. In many Asian countries, where grains, vegetables, and fish make up most of the diet, the consumption of fat is relatively low, and the rates of heart disease are low as well. It's been reported, however, that as these countries and the eating habits of their populations become more "westernized," the rates of heart disease and diabetes are increasing.

There's no question that many of us need to eat less fat, but how much less? What does thirty percent of total daily calories mean? First you need to know how many calories you need each day. If you aren't sure, follow the directions on page 19 to determine your total daily calories, then follow the steps below.

Step 1. Multiply your total daily calories by thirty percent, or 0.30. For example, if you need 1500 calories per day, multiply 1500 by 0.30 to determine how many fat calories you may eat in one day: 1500 x 0.30 = 450 total calories from fat.

Step 2. Divide the daily calories from fat by nine to determine how many grams of fat you can have in a day, because one gram of fat provides nine calories. Continuing with our example: 450 ÷ 9 = 50 total grams of fat.

Step 3. To determine how much saturated fat you may have, multiply your total daily calories by ten percent, or 0.10. For example, multiply 1500 by 0.10 percent to determine how many saturated fat calories you may eat in one day: 1500 x 0.10 = 150 calories from saturated fat. Divide the calories from saturated fat by nine to determine the grams of saturated fat you may have: 150 ÷ 9 = 17 grams of saturated fat (approximately).

Remember, you must include the grams or calories from saturated fat as part of, not in addition to, your total daily fat grams or calories. In our example, you would be able to eat a total of fifty grams of fat, and seventeen of those fifty grams could be from saturated fat.

How do you know when you've eaten the recommended amount of fat? You count, just as you do when you're monitoring the calories you consume. Fat grams, saturated fat grams, and calories from fat per serving appear on the Nutrition Facts panels on packaged foods, and many supermarkets display Nutrition Facts for meats, produce, and other foods that are not packaged with labels. Also, if you have the exchange information for a food, such as from the lists in this book, you can multiply the fat exchanges by five to determine the grams of fat per serving. (One fat exchange has five grams of fat.) One caution: Be sure to count the fat grams or calories from fat for *all* the foods you eat throughout the day including "hidden" fat such as the fat in meat or sweets and to keep the total fat calories at or under thirty percent of your total daily calories.

The following table shows the maximum recommended calories from fat, total fat grams, and saturated fat grams for various total calorie amounts. These are *maximum* recommended amounts; you may eat less than the recommended amounts of fat and saturated fat, but you should try not to eat more.

Total Calories	Calories from Fat	Total Fat Grams	Saturated Fat Grams
1200	360	40	13
1500	450	50	17
1800	540	60	20
2000	600	66	22
2200	660	73	24
2500	750	83	28
2800	840	93	31
3000	900	100	33
3500	1050	117	39

All About Food Fats

Dietary fats come from both plant and animal foods. They are an essential part of the diet and a major source of energy (calories). Dietary fat contributes more than twice as many calories as equal amounts (by weight) of either protein or carbohydrates. All types of fat contribute nine calories per gram.

Fatty acids are the building blocks of fat, and there are three kinds of fatty acids—saturated, monounsaturated, and polyunsaturated. A food is classified as contributing saturated or unsaturated fat to the diet based on the type of fatty acids it contains in the largest amount. Saturated fatty acids are solid at room temperature, and monounsaturated and polyunsaturated fatty acids are liquid at room temperature.

Saturated fats raise blood cholesterol levels. When substituted for saturated fats, monounsaturated fats may help to lower blood cholesterol and triglyceride levels. Although polyunsaturated fats also help lower blood cholesterol levels, some may lower HDL-cholesterol the "good" cholesterol as well. Special kinds of polyunsaturated fats called *omega-3 fatty acids* that are found in cold-water fish, such as mackerel, perch, cod, salmon, tuna, and

Note: Generally, fat should not be restricted in the diets of infants and toddlers below two years of age. After the age of two, total fat intake can be gradually decreased so that by five years of age no more than thirty percent of a child's daily calories are from fat. As calories from fat are decreased, these calories should be replaced by eating more grain products, fruits, vegetables, low-fat dairy products, and lean protein-rich foods (lean meat, poultry, fish, or dried beans).

sole, and in some fish oils, have a beneficial effect on blood triglycerides. The coronary heart disease rate is low in countries where
such fish is eaten often, even if the total fat intake is high. Because
of this, it's recommended that we eat fish two or more times a week.

Hydrogenation is a process that changes fatty acids from liquid to more solid forms at room temperature. Hydrogenation is
used to extend the shelf life of some products, but it also makes an
oil more saturated. Partially hydrogenated vegetable oils, such as
those in many margarine products and shortenings, contain a particular form of fat known as trans-fatty acids. Trans-fatty acids raise
blood cholesterol levels, although not as much as saturated fat.

Type of Fat	Origin	Some Sources
Saturated	Animal and Plant	Meat Cheese Butter Hardened shortenings Milk-fat dairy products Lard Coconut oil Palm oil Palm kernel oil
Monounsaturated	Animal and Plant	Canola oil Olive oil Peanut oil Avocados Most nuts
Polyunsaturated	Plant	Cottonseed oil Corn oil Safflower oil Sunflower oil Soybean oil Margarine

Tips for Reducing Fat in Your Diet

- Eat smaller and fewer meat servings. Most adults should limit total meat intake to about six ounces per day. Some women may need only four to five ounces a day. People on meal plans of more than 2000 calories may be able to have up to eight ounces of meat a day.

- Use lean meat exchanges whenever possible. Choose two or three servings of lean fish, poultry, meats, or other protein-rich foods, such as beans, daily. Today, many lower-fat and reduced-fat meat choices are available. Look for luncheon meats that have three or fewer grams of fat per ounce. See chapter 14 for a listing of lean meat choices.

- Choose high-fat meat exchanges no more than three times a week. Regular luncheon meats and other processed meats, frankfurters, wieners, sausage, bacon, and prime cuts of meat are high-fat meat choices.

- Avoid adding extra fat in the preparation of foods. Cook away as much fat as possible by baking, broiling, or roasting. When frying or sautéing foods, use nonfat cooking spray or a small amount of vegetable oil. If pan frying meat, drain the fat as it cooks out; if meat remains in the fat while cooking, the fat is reabsorbed by the meat.

- Chill gravies, soups, or stews until the fat hardens. Remove the fat layer, then re-heat and serve.

- Drink skim or 1% milk.

- Use plain nonfat yogurt (2 tablespoons = less than 20 calories) instead of sour cream (2 tablespoons = 50 calories) or mayonnaise (2 tablespoons = 200 calories) as a condiment or in recipes for dips and salad dressings.

- Choose cheeses that have five or fewer grams of fat per ounce.

- Use margarine instead of butter, but be careful of amounts. The calories in margarine and butter are the same, but because butter contains more saturated fatty acids than margarine, margarine is recommended. Look for margarine that lists a liquid oil such as corn, safflower, or soybean oil as the first ingredient. A soft or tub margarine is a better choice than solid or stick margarine.

- Choose low-fat or fat-free salad dressings. One tablespoon of a low-fat or fat-free salad dressing may have less than twenty calories and be considered a "free" food; two to three table-spoons is one fat exchange. If you prefer regular dressings, be very careful of the amount. One tablespoon is one fat exchange.
- Substitute nonfat dry milk or condensed skim milk for cream or non-dairy creamers. When using nonfat dry milk in hot beverages, allow the beverage to cool for a few minutes so the powder will dissolve without a curdled appearance. Non-dairy creamers contain about twenty calories per one-half ounce of liquid or one and a half teaspoons powder. One portion may be considered "free" or equivalent to one-half fat exchange. However, these products are usually made from palm or coconut oils or other hydrogenated vegetable oils, which are saturated fats. If you use a whitener only once or twice a day, the amount of fat consumed will not be signif-icant. But if you drink a significant amount of coffee each day and whiten it with a non-dairy creamer, you may be con-suming a considerable amount of saturated fat.
- Try some of the many light or fat-free sour creams, mayon-naise, and salad dressings on the market. They are made by using fat substitutes which have one to four calories per gram (rather than nine calories per gram of fat).

Fat Replacers: Problem or Panacea?

Ingredients: *cultured sour cream, skim milk, whey protein concen-trate, water, food starch-modified, lactic acid, maltodextrin, cellulose gum, potassium sorbate (a preservative), agar, vitamin A palmitate.*

Ingredients: *water, soybean oil, sugar, vinegar, food starch-modi-fied, salt, starch, cellulose gel (microcrystalline cellulose), sodium caseinate, mustard flour, egg white, xanthan gum, spice, paprika, natural flavor, beta carotene (color).*

Have you ever wondered what some of the ingredients *are* in the foods you buy? Well if you eat many light or reduced-calorie foods, at least part of the mystery is about to be solved—fat replacers.

The use of fat replacers in food manufacturing is growing rapidly as companies strive to give consumers what they want—good-tasting foods without the fat. More and more products are being made using fat replacers, and more and more fat replacers are being developed.

This is good for consumers. We now have many low-fat and reduced-calorie foods to choose from in the supermarket. Used wisely as part of a plan of healthy eating, these foods can help you reduce the fat and calories you consume while allowing you to eat foods you like.

But fat replacers are not the ultimate answer. These foods still have calories, and the danger of overeating looms large. When we are eating a healthy, low-fat food, there is a tendency to think we can have as much as we want. Many people end up consuming more calories by eating a large serving of a low-fat food than they would eating a normal serving of the regular food.

We can look at the use of sugar substitutes as an example. Sugar substitutes have been on the market since the early 1950s, yet sugar consumption has not decreased. Since 1965 sugar consumption has risen to about fourteen percent. The use of artificial sweeteners has more than doubled in that same time.

This is a good lesson as we continue to use products that contain fat replacers. Neither our personal health nor the health of our population will be improved by the indiscriminate use of foods containing fat replacers or by the potential increase in fat consumption that could accompany such use. However, when used wisely these foods can help us stay on track with our health and dietary goals.

The following chart lists fat replacers currently being used in food products, along with some that are under development. You may see these terms on food labels. Foods in which you are likely to find fat replacers also are noted in the table. (See appendix 2 for more about fat replacers.)

Fat Replacers

Terms you will see on food labels:	Foods you will find them in:
Made from carbohydrate	
Maltodextrin, corn syrup solids, hydrolyzed corn starch, modified food starch, polydextrose	Frozen desserts, cheese, baked goods, sauces, dressings, sour cream, yogurt, baked bread, meats, poultry
Pectin, carrageenan, sugar beet fiber or powder, cellulose gel, locust bean gum, xanthan gum, guar gum	Yogurt, sour cream, salad dressings, bakery products, frozen desserts, cheese spreads, sauces
Hydrogenated starch hydrolysate (HSH), hydrogenated glucose syrup, sorbitol, maltitol syrup, polydextrose	Baked goods, confections, chewing gum, frozen dairy desserts, gelatins, puddings, sauces, salad dressings, meat-based products
Made from protein	
Microparticulated egg white and milk protein, whey protein concentrate	Cheese, butter, mayonnaise, salad dressings, sour cream, bakery products, spreads
Made from fat	
Caprenin, Olestra, Salatrim, others being developed	Salatrim—chocolate, confections, cookies, crackers
	Olestra—savory snack foods, chips, crackers

Table adapted from "Fat Replacers: Their Use in Foods and Role in Diabetes Medical Nutrition Therapy," *Diabetes Care*, volume 19, number 11, November 1996.

Have you figured out what products the ingredient lists at the beginning of this section are from? The first is a light sour cream, and the second is a reduced-calorie salad dressing. Can you pick out which ingredients are fat replacers?

Fat replacers are making it possible to include many foods in a healthy diet that we may not have been able to include in the past, but they are not a magic potion for weight control or for healthy eating. How helpful they are depends on how you use them. A balanced, low-fat diet including a variety of foods and an eye toward portion control will still give you the best results.

In Summary

Making changes in your eating and cooking habits to help lower fat intake is good for you, and it's good for your family. Everyone can benefit from eating a low-fat diet. But don't try to do it all at once. Focus on making gradual changes that can last a lifetime. You can still have the occasional ice-cream cone or cookie; and you can do it without guilt when you know you are eating a healthy, low-fat diet every day.

CHAPTER 5

Sugar, Salt, and Fiber

When we think of healthy eating, we automatically think of fat, but other factors also contribute to a diet that promotes health. Just like fat, sugar and salt need to be monitored and kept at healthy levels in the diet. Most of us eat more sugar and salt than we need. Fiber, on the other hand, is beneficial to health, and many of us could use more. This chapter explains why diets low in sugar and salt and high in fiber are beneficial, and it offers tips for making healthy changes in your eating habits that will help decrease the sugar and salt and increase the fiber in your diet.

Sugar

Although humans have no inborn craving or urge for fat or salt, we naturally like sweetness. Animals too, with the exception of cats, have a "sweet tooth." However, many humans feed their sweet tooth so well that they crave unhealthy levels of sweetness.

Sugar occurs naturally in some foods, such as fruit, that are good foods to include in a healthy diet. The problem is added sugars, which contribute calories but no real nutritional advantage. Added sugars typically come from soft drinks, candy, jams, jellies, syrups, and table sugar added to foods like coffee or cereal. Added sugars also come from foods such as sweetened yogurts, chocolate milk, canned or frozen fruit with heavy syrup, cakes, pies, and cookies.

Although sugar has not been shown to be a risk factor for any serious health problems, it still makes good sense for everyone to use added sugars in moderation. The Food and Drug Administration estimates that Americans consume about forty-three pounds of added sugars per person per year, or about eleven percent of our total calories. This amounts to about four tablespoons per day. A diet with large amounts of sugar can have too many calories and too few nutrients for many people and can contribute to tooth decay. This chapter will give you tips on how to reduce sugar in your diet.

Added sugars are a special concern for people with diabetes. Sugar is a carbohydrate, and foods that contain significant amounts of added sugars are generally high in total carbohydrate as well as calories. Both factors contribute to elevated blood glucose levels. People with diabetes can eat foods that contain added sugars, but they must be careful of the amounts and must substitute correctly for them in their meal plans.

Added sugars and sweeteners are sometimes called nutritive sweeteners because they contribute calories. Common added sugars include white sugar, brown sugar, raw sugar, corn syrup, honey, and molasses. But there are other sugars and sweeteners added to baked and processed foods that may not be as familiar to you. Many sugars and sweeteners have names that end in "ose." Sugar alcohols, another form of sugar used for sweetening foods, have names that end in "ol." The following are some of the more common sugars and sweeteners which you may see on food labels. A complete list with brief explanations appears in appendix 3.

Common Sugars and Sweeteners

Dextrin	High fructose corn syrup	Mannitol
Dextrose		Polyols
Fructose	Hydrogenated starch hydrolysates	Sorbitol
Fruit juice concentrate	Invert sugar	Sorghum
Galactose	Lactose	Sucrose
	Maltose	Turbinado sugar
		Xylitol

Sugar Substitutes

Sugar substitutes are sometimes referred to as non-nutritive sweeteners, or low- or non-caloric sweeteners, because they contribute few or no calories. They are intensely sweet, so only very small amounts are needed to sweeten food products. Although some sugar substitutes contribute calories, they are usually used in such small amounts in manufacturing that the contribution to caloric intake is not significant.

Food manufacturers have a variety of sugar substitutes to choose from in formulating new products. Each sweetener can be used in the products and processes for which it is best suited. This allows for more choices in low-calorie food products, which is a plus for consumers.

The following are sugar substitutes available for use in the United States and some that are currently being reviewed for approval by the Food and Drug Administration (FDA).

Saccharin. Although saccharin has been used for about eighty years, it was designated by the FDA in 1977 as a possible cancer-causing agent. This was due to a study that showed a probability of inducing cancer in rats with a saccharin intake equal to about 800 cans of diet soda a day. There is no evidence to suggest that saccharin causes cancer in humans.

Aspartame. Aspartame is a combination of two amino acids (aspartic acid and phenylalanine) that when combined are intensely sweet. It is marketed as a tabletop sweetener called Equal®. Aspartame also is used in a variety of food products under the brand names of NutraSweet®, NutraTaste®, and others.

Before it was approved for use in foods, aspartame underwent more than 100 scientific studies in over twenty years. According to the FDA, "few compounds have withstood such detailed testing and repeated close scrutiny." The only documented harm from aspartame is in people with a very rare inherited disease called phenylketonuria (PKU), and a warning to people with PKU appears on all foods containing aspartame.

Acesulfame-K. Acesulfame-K is a manmade sweetener with a high degree of stability when exposed to heat. It is used primarily for tabletop sweeteners and marketed in the United States and Canada under the brand names of Sunette®, SweetOne®, or Swiss Sweet™. Acesulfame-K has been reviewed and determined to be safe by regulatory authorities in more than twenty countries. Its safety is supported by more than ninety studies conducted over fifteen years.

Sucralose. Approved for use in Canada and Australia, sucralose is the first sugar substitute made from sugar. It has no calories and can be used virtually anywhere sugar can be used, including in cooking. Sucralose can be used in baking as well, as long as it is in recipes developed specifically for its use. Sucralose retains sweetness over long storage periods and at elevated temperatures. Extensive studies have been conducted and evaluated to show and support that sucralose is safe for humans to use. In the United States, sucralose is still under review by the FDA.

Cyclamate. Cyclamates were removed from the market in 1973, principally on the basis of one experiment showing that its use at very high doses was related to the development of bladder tumors in rats. However, seventy-five subsequent studies have failed to demonstrate that cyclamate causes cancer. The FDA is currently reviewing a petition for re-approval.

Alitame. Alitame is formed from the amino acids aspartic acid and alanine. It is stable at high temperatures and would be suitable for use in a wide variety of products such as beverages, tabletop sweeteners, frozen desserts, and baked goods. Alitame has been shown to be safe in more than fifteen studies, but approval is delayed in the United States.

The FDA sets an accepted daily intake (ADI) for food additives such as sugar substitutes. The ADI is the amount that is determined to be safe for humans to consume on a daily basis over a lifetime without adverse effects. It is about $\frac{1}{100}$ of the amount tested and shown to have no toxic effect in animals.

The ADI is reported as an amount per kilogram (2.2 pounds equals 1 kg) of body weight. For example, 50 mg/kg is the ADI for aspartame. For a 150-pound (70 kg) person, this represents twenty twelve-ounce cans of diet soft drinks sweetened with aspartame or ninety-seven packets of Equal®. For a fifty-pound (23 kg) child, it takes seven diet soft drinks or thirty-two packets of Equal® to reach ADI levels. As you can see, the ADI includes a very generous safety factor.

Tips for Reducing Sugar in Your Diet

- Substitute water or fruit juice for soft drinks. Soft drinks are the largest single source of sugar in the diet. The sugar in one twelve-ounce can of cola supplies 145 calories or the equivalent of nine to ten teaspoons of sugar.

- Cut back on commercial baked goods such as pastries, sweet rolls, and cookies, which are the second biggest source of sugar after soft drinks.

- Eat fruit or low-fat frozen yogurt for dessert.

- Reduce the amount of sugar in recipes. You can often use one-half to one-third the amount called for without affecting taste.

- Use vanilla, cinnamon, or nutmeg to add flavor without adding calories.

- Look for sugar-free foods that have twenty calories or less and use them as "free foods."
- Use low-sugar or light jam instead of syrup on pancakes and waffles. An average one-quarter cup serving of pancake syrup has as much sugar as is found in four to five apples or oranges.
- Use sugar substitutes in place of sugar to sweeten beverages and foods.
- Avoid eating candy bars as snacks. One candy bar has as much sugar as a half pound of apples.

Salt

When we hear the terms "salt" or "sodium," we usually think of table salt. Table salt is composed of two minerals—sodium and chloride. About one-third of the sodium in our diets comes straight from the salt shaker, so cutting down on table salt is a good way to cut down on sodium. But what about the other two-thirds? A good bit of it comes from processed foods, and this is another area where changes can be made to reduce salt.

Although some sodium is necessary for the body to function, we consume far more than we need. The body requires only about 220 milligrams of sodium per day, or the equivalent of one-tenth teaspoon of salt. (One teaspoon of salt contains 2300 milligrams of sodium.) Yet the average daily intake is 4000 to 5000 milligrams of sodium, or two to three teaspoons of salt. We could easily get all the sodium we need, even if we never added salt in processing or cooking food.

We are all encouraged to cut back on our sodium (salt) intake. A diet high in salt is associated with high blood pressure (hypertension), heart disease, and kidney disease. It's recommended that we try to keep our sodium intake to less than 3000 milligrams per day, or about 800 to 1000 milligrams per meal. This is especially important for people who have a family history of high blood pressure. If you have high blood pressure yourself, you need to limit your sodium intake to less than 2400 milligrams per day, or less than 700 milligrams per meal.

Everyone has individual needs. Your doctor or dietitian can help you determine what health problems you have or are at risk for and how much sodium you should be using. The following chart lists recommended sodium intake for various medical risks.

Recommended Sodium Intake

Health Factors	Sodium Level	Guidelines
Healthy person who wants to control sodium intake for disease prevention	3000 milligrams per day	Eliminate use of table salt. Seldom use convenience foods with more than 800 milligrams of sodium per serving.
Mild hypertension Mild heart disease Mild fluid retention	2400 milligrams per day	Eliminate use of table salt. Use minimal amounts of salt in cooking. Avoid foods containing more than 400 milligrams of sodium per serving.
Moderate to severe hypertension Kidney disease Heart disease Moderate to severe fluid retention	1000–2000 milligrams per day	Eliminate use of table salt. Use minimal amounts of salt in cooking. Eat only foods with less than 140 milligrams of sodium per serving.

Tips for Reducing Salt in Your Diet

- Add little or no salt to foods at the table. Leave the salt shaker in the cupboard, and pass the pepper!

- Taste foods before deciding if they really need salt.

- Cook with little or no added salt. When cooking pastas, vegetables, and cereals you can easily skip the salt without losing much flavor, and you can use half the salt called for in many recipes. In some recipes, you can leave the salt out altogether. However many baked recipes, especially those with yeast, require salt for the recipe to work.

- Read food labels and look for foods with 400 milligrams or less sodium per serving and 800 milligrams or less sodium per convenience dinner or entrée. (See chapter 6 for more about food labels.)

- Avoid high-sodium meats like ham, bacon, sausage, and cold cuts.

- Rinse canned foods with fresh water to reduce the sodium content. Rinsing the contents of a can of tuna for one minute will wash away about three-fourths of the sodium. Almost half the sodium can be removed from canned vegetables by rinsing for one minute and heating the vegetables in tap water instead of the canning liquid.

- Use herbs and spices instead of salt. Begin by using no more than one or two herbs or spices at a time. As a general rule, use one-quarter teaspoon of dried herbs or three to four teaspoons of the fresh herb for every four servings of food. Add herbs or seasonings to soups or stews during the last hour of cooking to retain flavor. In cold dressings, dips, or marinades, add herbs and spices several hours before serving to "blend" the flavors.

- Try salt-free herb blends.

- Limit use of salt-based condiments such as soy sauce, steak sauce, catsup, and Worcestershire sauce, or use low-salt varieties.

- Substitute onion and garlic powders for onion and garlic salts.

- Choose low-sodium or lower-salt crackers, snacks, and soups.

- Limit use of fast foods. A quick rule of thumb is to limit your sodium intake at one fast-food meal to one-third of your total sodium allowance for the day. If you exceed the recommended amount, you need to be especially careful of your food choices during the rest of the day.

Fiber

Fiber is the structural part (or cell wall) of fruits, vegetables, grains, nuts, and legumes that can't be digested or broken down in the human digestive tract or absorbed into the bloodstream. There are two types of dietary fiber—insoluble and soluble—and each has specific health benefits.

Insoluble fiber gives plants structure. It's called insoluble because it does not dissolve in water. It adds bulk to the diet and has a laxative effect on the digestive system. You usually feel full after eating foods containing insoluble fiber as well. Common sources are wheat and corn bran, whole grains, nuts, and some vegetables and fruits.

Soluble fibers form a gel because they are soluble in water. They include fibers found in oats, legumes, barley, seeds, and some fruits and vegetables, particularly those with edible peels and seeds. Most soluble fibers are found within plant cells. The gummy texture of oat bran and the mushy center of a cooked kidney bean reflect the soluble fiber content and the ability of soluble fibers to soak up water. Soluble fibers help lower blood cholesterol levels, especially when included in a low-fat diet.

Mostly Insoluble Fiber	Both Soluble and Insoluble Fiber	Mostly Soluble Fiber
Wheat bran	Oat bran	Citrus fruits
Whole wheat products	Whole-grain oats	Pectin
Corn bran	Barley	Carrageenan
Brown rice	Navy beans	Guar gum
Rice bran	Soybeans	
Bananas	Kidney beans	
Cauliflower	Apples	
Nuts	Potatoes	
Lentils	Broccoli	
Green beans	Carrots	
Green peas		

Studies indicate a positive relationship between a high-fiber diet and decreased risk of disease. It has been difficult, however, to separate the effects of fiber from other dietary and lifestyle factors that play a role in health. For example, people who eat more fiber tend also to eat less fat, and low-fat diets also contribute to good health.

The most well-established health benefit of a high-fiber diet is in the treatment and prevention of constipation. Large amounts of insoluble fibers increase stool bulk and draw water into the large intestine. The result is a larger, softer stool that exerts less pressure on the colon walls and is eliminated more quickly. This is one reason that the National Cancer Institute and the American Cancer Society have recommended low-fat diets generous in dietary fiber to reduce the risk of some cancers. If food contains carcinogens (cancer-causing agents), fiber speeds up the transit time of stools through the digestive system, thus reducing exposure of the intestinal wall to those substances.

Diets rich in soluble fibers have been shown to lower total blood cholesterol levels and LDL-cholesterol in people with both high and normal blood cholesterol levels. But perhaps the most important benefit of foods containing fiber is that they also contain important vitamins and minerals.

Getting Enough Fiber

Estimates currently indicate that our average dietary fiber intake is between ten to thirty grams a day; men average nineteen grams a day and women thirteen grams. Major health organizations, including the American Diabetes Association, advise a daily intake of twenty to thirty-five grams of fiber a day. The Diet and Health report of the National Academy of Sciences goes one step further by specifying a daily intake of five or more servings of fruits and vegetables and six or more servings of whole-grain breads and cereals and legumes. Fiber supplements are not recommended as a way to meet dietary guidelines because they usually do not contain large amounts of dietary fiber, nor do they have all the nutrients that accompany fiber in foods.

It is important not to go overboard with an immediate leap from a low-fiber intake to recommended levels. Increasing fiber too rapidly can cause flatulence (gas), cramping, diarrhea, or bloating. Undesirable side effects may be avoided by gradually adding fiber to the diet along with adequate amounts of liquids.

Tips for Increasing Fiber in Your Diet

- Switch from white bread to whole-grain varieties. Choose products made from stone ground flour, 100% whole wheat, or other whole grain flours. They should be the first ingredient on the label. "Brown-colored" breads contain little or no whole grain, just molasses for coloring. If the label says "wheat flour" it usually refers to bleached, white flour.

- Select whole fresh fruit and vegetables instead of juices. Eat the skin of cleaned fruit (such as apples), membranes (such as oranges), and seeds (such as strawberries). Eat more raw and slightly cooked vegetables such as corn, peas, beans, legumes, and potatoes with the skin. The stems and leaves of salad greens and broccoli are also fibrous. Don't throw away these good fiber sources. Add dry beans and peas to soups, stews, and casseroles. Use these legumes as main dishes, along with whole wheat pasta.

- Choose high-fiber, low-fat snacks. Snack on vegetables, fruit, air-popped popcorn, and cereals, rather than cakes, cookies, and chocolate.

One cautionary note: If you add extra calories by adding high-fiber foods to your daily eating instead of substituting them for other food choices, you will probably gain weight. To save calories, trim your intake of high-fat, high-calorie foods. Chapter 4 gives tips for cutting the fat in your diet.

In Summary

Generally, the more unprocessed a food is, the more nutritious it is. Foods with less added sugar and salt are better choices than foods containing large amounts of sugar and salt. And by choosing foods in their more natural state instead of highly refined foods, you will benefit from the fiber and the valuable vitamins and minerals high-fiber foods contain. This all adds up to a healthy diet.

PART TWO

Using Exchanges in Everyday Life

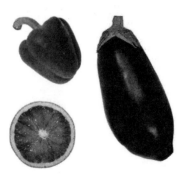

CHAPTER 6

Using Food Labels

Food labels are a great source of information that can help you choose healthy foods and fit them into your meal plan. Information displayed on food labels is regulated by two agencies of the government: the Food and Drug Administration (FDA) and the United States Department of Agriculture (USDA). The FDA regulates the labeling of all packaged food products and the ingredients that are added to foods, while the USDA regulates the labeling of meat and poultry products.

The Nutrition Facts Panel

The Nutrition Facts panel on food labels provides information about calories, fat, saturated fat, cholesterol, carbohydrate, sodium, protein, iron, calcium, and vitamins A and C. Regulations require Nutrition Facts panels to be included on most packaged foods. The exceptions are foods that have no nutritional significance to the diet (such as plain coffee, tea, and spices); foods sold in very small packages; and food prepared on-site and intended for immediate consumption, such as deli and bakery items. Nutrition information for fresh fruits and vegetables and raw meat and fish often is displayed at the point of purchase.

An example of a Nutrition Facts panel is shown on the next page. As you read Nutrition Facts information, keep in mind that some packaged foods require the addition of ingredients during preparation, such as butter, milk, or eggs. In this case, the nutrition information may be for the product as packaged, but not necessarily for the food as it is prepared. Look closely at the Nutrition Facts. Products that give nutrition information for the food "as prepared" will state this plainly. If this is not the case and the information provided is for the packaged contents only, you will need to make allowances for ingredients that you add during preparation.

The first line under the title, Nutrition Facts, lists the serving size, which reflects the amount commonly eaten as one serving.

Nutrition Facts

Serving Size 1 cup (228g)
Servings Per Container 2

Amount Per Serving

Calories 260 Calories from Fat 120

	% Daily Value*
Total Fat 13g	**20%**
Saturated Fat 5g	**25%**
Cholesterol 30mg	**10%**
Sodium 660mg	**28%**
Total Carbohydrate 31g	**10%**
Dietary Fiber 0g	**0%**
Sugar 5g	
Protein 5g	

Vitamin A 4%	•	Vitamin C 2%
Calcium 15%	•	Iron 4%

* Percent daily values are based on a 2,000 calorie diet. Your daily values may be higher or lower depending on your calorie needs:

	Calories:	2,000	2,500
Total Fat	Less than	65g	80g
Sat Fat	Less than	20g	25g
Cholesterol	Less than	300mg	300mg
Sodium	Less than	2400mg	2400mg
Total Carbohydrate		300g	375g
Dietary Fiber		25g	30g

Calories per gram:
Fat 9 • Carbohydrate 4 • Protein 4

Similar food products have similar serving sizes, making it easier to compare the nutritional content of different products. Serving sizes are listed in common household and metric measures—1 cup (228 g), for example—and the rest of the Nutrition Facts information is based on this serving size. If you eat double the serving size, you also consume twice the calories, fat, and other nutrients.

The serving size used to calculate Nutrition Facts information may be different from the serving size used to calculate the exchange value for the exchange lists. For example, the serving size on the Nutrition Facts panel for orange juice is eight ounces (1 cup or 240 milliliters), and the serving size in the Fruit List is four ounces (½ cup or 120 milliliters). If you drink one cup of orange juice, you must count it as two fruit exchanges (or two carbohydrate choices).

Calories for the serving size are listed along with the number of calories from fat. The nutrients listed next are those most important to your health. The value listed for total carbohydrate includes the dietary fiber and sugars listed below it. Sugars include those that occur naturally, such as lactose in milk and fructose in fruits, and those added to the food, such as table sugar, corn syrup, and dextrose. Only two vitamins, A and C, and two minerals, calcium and iron, are required on the the Nutrition Facts panel. However, a food company can voluntarily list other vitamins and minerals that are in the food.

The % Daily Value column shows how a food fits into a 2000-calorie diet. These percentages are based on the reference numbers for daily fat, cholesterol, sodium, and carbohydrate shown at the bottom of the Nutrition Facts panel. These numbers are set by the FDA and are based on current nutrition recommendations. Some panels list the daily values for daily diets of both 2000 and 2500 calories. These numbers are for reference only; your own nutrient needs depend on your total daily calories and may be less than or more than the values on the panel.

Making Healthy Food Choices

The Nutrition Facts panel provides the information you need to make healthy food choices and to fit a variety of foods into your meal plan. There are three main items on the panel that will help you do this: serving size, calories, and fat. Sodium content also is important for people who need to monitor their sodium intake, such as people with high blood pressure. (People with diabetes need to pay close attention to the carbohydrates in their food choices, and this is discussed on page 22.)

Serving size. Dishing up a reasonable serving of a food and knowing how to count *that* amount of *that* food in your meal plan is critical. Many people have difficulty in this area because, unless you weigh or measure your food servings, your perception of how much you're eating may or may not be accurate. The key here is to remember that all the nutrition information on the Nutrition Facts panel is dependent on the serving size. If you misjudge how much of a food you're eating, you also will count it incorrectly in your meal plan. You must count the total amount of the food you eat. As mentioned earlier, the serving size given on the Nutrition Facts panel may be different from the serving size given in the exchange lists. In such cases, you need to make the appropriate adjustments when determining exchange values.

Calories. Most "diets" focus on calories as the guiding factor in determining what and how much to eat, so most of us know how to count calories. Calories are certainly an important part of any meal plan, but it's more important to get those calories from a variety of healthy foods. That's what your meal plan is designed to help you do. Use the calorie information on Nutrition Facts panels to determine whether to use the foods and how much to eat. Remember that a serving of a food or drink that supplies twenty calories or less is a free food. If it supplies more than twenty calories, you need to count it in your meal plan.

For most adults, a weight maintenance program is based on about 1800 to 2400 calories per day. This translates to about 600 to 800 calories at a meal. To lose weight, most adults need about 1500 to 1800 calories per day, or about 500 to 600 at each meal. Page 19 gives directions for determining your personal calorie needs.

Fat. We tend to blame everything on fat, and in fact large amounts of fat in the diet have been shown to contribute to a variety of health problems, from obesity to heart disease. We need to remember, though, that fat plays an important role in nutrition, and some fat is necessary for our bodies to function properly. Nevertheless, most of us eat too much fat.

Fat contributes about thirty percent of the calories in a healthy diet. It's impractical to expect, though, that you will meet this guideline at every meal or with every food you eat. For instance, most meat has more than thirty percent fat, and bread has much less. Also, many of us eat more fat at the evening meal than at other meals because more meat is usually eaten then. The guideline for fat is meant to help you look at what you eat over the course of a day, or even a week, and keep your fat intake at a healthy level overall. The fat information on Nutrition Facts panels, given in grams, is an important guide for making food choices that support your efforts to do this. The table on page 34 gives the recommended number of fat grams per day for various total daily calorie amounts.

The fat information on Nutrition Facts panels also is very helpful for choosing low-fat foods, particularly snack and convenience foods, that fit well into a healthy, low-fat diet. Foods with three grams or less fat per 100 calories are good choices. You can use the following table to convert fat grams into fat exchanges and to help you fit foods into your meal plan. However, if the food is a combination food that includes meat or a meat substitute such as cheese, some of the fat grams listed on the Nutrition Facts panel will be counted as part of the meat exchanges. In such cases, the fat grams do not convert directly into fat exchanges (see appendix 4).

Fat Grams	Fat Exchanges
0–2	–
3	½ fat
4–7	1 fat
8	1½ fat
9–12	2 fat
13	2½ fat
14–17	3 fat

Let's look at some Nutrition Facts panels and compare different food choices. The nutrient values of food exchanges appear on page 283.

Regular Potato Chips	**Reduced-Fat Potato Chips**	**Low-Fat Baked Potato Chips**
Serving Size 1 oz (17 chips)	Serving Size 1 oz (16 Chips)	Serving Size 1 oz (12 chips)
Calories 160	Calories 140	Calories 110
Total Fat 10 g	Total Fat 7 g	Total Fat 1.5 g
Total Carb 14 g	Total Carb 18 g	Total Carb 23 g
Protein 2 g	Protein 2 g	Protein 2 g

The Nutrition Facts tell you that potato chips contain carbohydrate, fat, and a little protein. You'll notice that the grams of carbohydrate increase as the grams of fat decrease. This is because the fat is replaced by carbohydrate-based fat replacers in the reduced-fat and low-fat potato chips. (See page 37 for more information about fat replacers.) The total calories decrease because carbohydrate supplies fewer calories than fat. Potatoes are on the Starch List, and one serving from this list has fifteen grams of carbohydrate and three grams of protein. One fat serving supplies five grams of fat. Divide the total carbohydrate grams by fifteen and the fat grams by five to determine how many carbohydrate and fat exchanges each food provides.

- One serving of the regular potato chips = 1 starch (1 carbohydrate choice) and 2 fat exchanges
- One serving of the reduced-fat potato chips = 1 starch (1 carbohydrate choice) and 1½ fat exchanges
- One serving of low-fat baked potato chips = 1½ starch exchanges (1½ carbohydrate choices)

Only the low-fat baked potato chips meet the low-fat guideline, and in fact they exceed it, so they are the best choice if you want to follow a low-fat diet. You could eat either of the other two varieties and fit the exchanges into your meal plan. It's just a matter of how you want to use your fat exchanges, or grams, and your calories. It's interesting to note that you could eat two servings (two ounces) of the low-fat baked potato chips and still get fewer calories and less fat than if you ate one serving (one ounce) of the regular potato chips. However, you would have to count the two servings as three starch exchanges and one half to one fat in your meal plan.

Regular Mayonnaise	Light Mayonnaise	Fat-Free Mayonnaise Dressing
Serving Size 1 Tbsp (14 g)	Serving Size 1 Tbsp (15 g)	Serving Size 1 Tbsp (16 g)
Calories 100	Calories 50	Calories 10
Total Fat 11 g	Total Fat 5 g	Total Fat 0 g
Total Carb 0 g	Total Carb 2 g	Total Carb 2 g
Protein 0 g	Protein 0 g	Protein 0 g

The Nutrition Facts tell you that mayonnaise contains fat and/or small amounts of carbohydrate. The carbohydrate in the second and third products is from a fat replacer. Mayonnaise is on the Fat List, and each serving on this list contains five grams of fat. Divide the grams of fat in the food by five to determine how many fat exchanges each food provides.

- One serving of the regular mayonnaise = 2 fat exchanges
- One serving of the light mayonnaise = 1 fat exchange
- One serving of the fat-free mayonnaise = 1 free food

Only the fat-free mayonnaise meets the low-fat guideline. It is the best choice for a healthy, low-fat diet. But since mayonnaise is a fat anyway, this choice may be governed largely by serving size. If one tablespoon of mayonnaise is enough and you have two fat exchanges to use, you can choose the regular mayonnaise. However, you may choose one of the reduced-fat products so that you can use more than one tablespoon or so you can use your fat exchanges in some other way.

The information on Nutrition Facts panels does help you choose low-fat foods, but you need to estimate exchanges for most of the foods you buy in order to fit the food into your meal plan. We have done that for you for many foods, and the information appears in the lists in this book. However, you also can use the information from the Nutrition Facts panel on any food to estimate the exchanges in a serving. See appendix 4 for directions on how to do this.

Nutrition Facts and Carbohydrate Counting

If you have diabetes, carbohydrate counting is a great way to add flexibility and variety to your meal planning, and the Nutrition Facts panel can help. The basics of carbohydrate counting and why it helps with blood glucose control are discussed on page 22. Here you will learn how to apply carbohydrate counting to making food choices. Remember, you still need to be aware of fat and protein in foods, so the information in the previous section is important for you as well.

Because your main goal in meal planning is to balance the food you eat, specifically the carbohydrate, with your insulin and physical activity, you need to focus on the carbohydrate information given on the Nutrition Facts panel. You can determine the number of carbohydrate "choices" provided by most food products using the "15-Gram Equation."

The 15-Gram Equation
15 grams of carbohydrate = 1 carbohydrate choice

For example, if the panel states that one serving is two oatmeal cookies and contains thirty grams of carbohydrate, you would count those two cookies as two carbohydrate choices (30 ÷ 15 = 2). However, if you ate four oatmeal cookies you would need to count them as four carbohydrate choices. You can ignore the grams of sugar listed on Nutrition Facts panels; sugar is included in the total grams of carbohydrate.

Of course, the number of grams of carbohydrate in foods is not always neatly divisible by fifteen, and carbohydrate counting is not an exact science. The chart below, which is based on the 15-Gram Equation, shows the relationship of carbohydrate grams to carbohydrate choices. Use it when you shop to determine quickly how to include the foods you like in your meal plan.

Carbohydrate Grams	Carbohydrate Choices
0–5	0
6–10	½
11–20	1
21–25	1½
26–35	2
36–40	2½
41–50	3
51–55	3½
56–65	4
66–70	4½
71–80	5

The number of carbohydrate choices for high-fiber foods, such as beans and some cereals, will not follow the 15-Gram Equation. This is because fiber is not digested or absorbed by the body but simply "passes through" without affecting blood glucose levels. This can be tricky when reading the Nutrition Facts panel because carbohydrate from fiber is included in the total carbohydrate listed. If there are more than five grams of dietary fiber in a food, subtract the grams of dietary fiber from the total grams of carbohydrate before calculating the carbohydrate choices.

Foods that contain sugar alcohols also require special consideration when using carbohydrate counting. If there are more than five grams of a sugar alcohol (sorbitol, mannitol, xylitol), subtract one-half the grams of sugar alcohol from the total grams of carbohydrate before calculating the carbohydrate choices.

Let's look at some examples of how the information on the Nutrition Facts panel can help you choose foods and fit them into your meal plan using carbohydrate counting.

Regular Syrup	Reduced-Calorie Syrup	Sugar-Free Syrup
Serving Size ¼ cup (60 ml)	Serving Size ¼ cup (60 ml)	Serving Size ¼ cup (60 ml)
Calories 200	Calories 100	Calories 20
Total Fat 0 g	Total Fat 0 g	Total Fat 0 g
Total Carb 57 g	Total Carb 26 g	Total Carb 9 g
Sugars 38 g	Sugars 25 g	Sugars 0 g
		Sorbitol 8 g
Protein 0 g	Protein 0 g	Protein 0 g

The Nutrition Facts show that syrup contains primarily carbohydrate. Syrup is on the Other Carbohydrates List because it is mostly sugar. Foods on the Other Carbohydrates List contain fifteen grams of carbohydrate per serving. Divide the grams of carbohydrate on the panel by fifteen to determine how many exchanges one serving of each product provides. If the answer is a fraction, round to the nearest one half.

- One serving of the regular syrup = 4 other carbohydrate exchanges (4 carbohydrate choices)
- One serving of the reduced-calorie syrup = 2 other carbohydrate exchanges (2 carbohydrate choices)
- One serving of the sugar-free syrup = 1 free food (20 calories or less per serving)

The sugar-free syrup may be the best choice. However, if you prefer the regular syrup because of taste, you need to count it in your meal plan. If you don't have three to four carbohydrate choices to use, you'll have to have less than one serving. One third of the one-quarter cup serving, about one tablespoon, would equal one carbohydrate choice.

Cherry Fruit-on-the-Bottom Low-Fat Yogurt

Serving Size 1 container 8 oz (227 g)

Calories 240

Total Fat 3 g

Total Carb 46 g

Sugars 44 g

Protein 9 g

Light Cherry Nonfat Yogurt with Aspartame

Serving Size 1 container 8 oz (227 g)

Calories 100

Total Fat 0 g

Total Carb 16 g

Sugars 12 g

Protein 8 g

These panels tell us that yogurt with fruit contains carbohydrate and protein. Yogurt is on the Milk List and fruit is on the Fruit List. One milk exchange has twelve grams of carbohydrate, eight grams of protein, and zero to three grams of fat. One fruit exchange has fifteen grams of carbohydrate.

• One container of the yogurt with fruit on the bottom = 1 milk exchange and 2 fruit exchanges (3 carbohydrate choices)

• One container of the light cherry yogurt sweetened with aspartame = 1 milk exchange (1 carbohydrate choice)

The use of a sugar substitute in the second yogurt reduces the amount of carbohydrate significantly. The use of a fat replacer eliminates fat in the product as well. Calories are also reduced significantly. The amount of carbohydrate in the first yogurt is close to what is usually planned for an entire meal; the second yogurt provides an amount of carbohydrate appropriate for a snack.

Label Terms and Health Claims

In addition to the information on the Nutrition Facts panel, the FDA and the USDA also regulate which descriptive or health terms food manufacturers can put on a food package or label. In order to be considered "light," or "low calorie," for example, a product must meet certain criteria. This ensures that if you buy a product with a label that reads "low fat," then it really *is* low fat. Common food label terms and their meanings are listed below.

If a label reads . . .	then the product has . . .
Free	
Fat-free	½ gram or less fat per serving
Sugar-free	½ gram or less sugar per serving
Calorie-free	5 calories or less per serving
Low	
Low-fat	3 grams or less fat per serving
Low-calorie	40 calories or less per serving
No sugar added	No sugar added during processing, including ingredients that contain sugar, such as fruit juice
Reduced	
Reduced or less fat	At least 25% less fat than the regular food
Reduced or less sugar	At least 25% less sugar than the regular food
Reduced or fewer calories	At least 25% fewer calories than the regular food
Light *or* Lite	⅓ less calories or 50% less fat than the regular product

Some food packages or labels also may carry health claims. A health claim is a label statement that establishes a relationship between a nutrient and a disease or health-related condition. An example would be claiming a food is beneficial in the prevention of cancer because it is high in fiber. Usually these claims aren't made directly on the food package; rather, the claim may be made in advertisements. A food must meet certain nutrient levels to make a health claim, and health claims must be approved by the FDA. The following are examples of health claims and the health condition to which each relates.

A label may say . . .	to establish a beneficial relationship to . . .
High in fiber	Cancer; heart disease
Low in fat, saturated fat, and cholesterol	Cancer; heart disease
Low in sodium	High blood pressure
High in calcium	Osteoporosis

Ingredients List

A food package or label is also required to show the list of ingredients used to make the food. All ingredients are listed in descending order by weight. The amount of each ingredient is weighed, and the ingredient that weighs the most is listed first. The ingredient that weighs the least is listed last. Ingredients that make up two percent or less of a food are listed at the end of the list in no particular order.

If you are trying to control your intake of fat, cholesterol, sodium, or other substances, ingredient lists are helpful in making appropriate food choices. For example, for good nutrition it's important to be aware of ingredients that are high in saturated fat. Some people also need to watch their sodium intake. Though fat and sodium content are listed on the Nutrition Facts panel, it can be very helpful to know which ingredients are supplying it. Some ingredients that are high in saturated fat or sodium are listed below.

High in Saturated Fat
Animal fat
Bacon
Beef fat
Butter
Chicken fat
Coconut oil
Hydrogenated shortening
Lard
Palm kernel oil
Palm oil

High in Sodium
Bouillon
Brine (salt and water)
Broth
Monosodium glutamate (MSG)
Salt
Sodium chloride
Soy sauce

Read ingredients lists as you shop and learn to spot ingredients you want to avoid. (See chapter 4 for information about reducing fat in your diet and chapter 5 for information about reducing salt in your diet.)

In Summary

The Nutrition Facts panel is the most helpful information on a food package or label. Remember to begin by noting the serving size, because all the other information on the Nutrition Facts panel is based on the serving size given. This panel tells you everything you need to know about the food in order to fit it into your meal plan.

CHAPTER 7

Cooking With Exchanges

Do you enjoy baking and cooking? If you do, there are many ways you can make the foods you prepare healthier. The final test for food preparation is always taste, but lowering fat, salt, or sugar or increasing fiber can help make your recipes easier to fit into a healthy meal plan. There are many ways to do this while keeping the good taste of the food.

Making Recipes Healthier

There are two basic ways to modify a recipe: change an ingredient or change a cooking technique. An example of changing an ingredient is sautéing vegetables in broth instead of in oil or butter. This reduces total fat and saturated fat. An example of changing a cooking technique is broiling a hamburger instead of frying it. This reduces fat because much of the fat drips into the broiling pan; fat is absorbed back into the food when foods are fried.

Besides substituting a healthier ingredient, you can modify ingredients by reducing them or eliminating them completely. Before deciding to do this, analyze the function of the ingredient carefully and make sure it is not necessary to the success of the final product. For example, the ratio of flour, salt, and baking powder in some baked foods is crucial in achieving the right texture. However, sugar often can be reduced without harm. Look for dispensable ingredients that are high in fat, sugar, or salt. Sometimes ingredients are added for appearance or because of habit and tradition and are not really needed.

Sugar substitutes sometimes can be used to lower sugar, calories, and carbohydrate in recipes, especially beverage recipes. The following will help you use sugar substitutes successfully.

- Sugar substitutes are generally not useful in baked desserts because sugar is required to produce a light and airy texture. Instead of using a sugar substitute, you can try to reduce the amount of sugar called for in the recipe.

- In some foods, aspartame (Equal®) or other sugar substitutes can be used to sweeten without sugar, however, it should not be added before cooking in the oven or on the range. Heat may cause aspartame to lose its sweetness, so add it after the cooking process when the food has cooled slightly.

- Liquid sugar substitutes can be added directly to food during preparation. Tablets may be crushed and stirred into a liquid mixture, or they may be dissolved first in a small amount of liquid called for in the recipe and then added to the rest of the mixture. Granulated sweeteners, including NutraSweet® Spoonful, may be added in the same way sugar would be added to cold or non-baked recipes.

- Acesulfame-K (SweetOne®) is stable to heat and therefore can be used in cooking and baking. For best results use recipes developed for use with SweetOne®, or experiment by substituting half the sugar called for in a recipe with the equivalent amount of SweetOne®.

The table on page 71 offers more ideas for making your favorite recipes healthier. It lists modifications and substitutions for lowering fat, sugar, and salt and for adding fiber when preparing foods at home. Your recipes will be healthier but still look and taste good.

Calculating Exchanges for Recipes

If you have recipes that you enjoy or that you have modified and make often, you may wish to know how many exchanges are in one serving so you can fit it into your meal plan. You can use two methods to convert your recipes to exchanges. Both use the information from the Common Baking and Cooking Ingredients table on page 73.

Method 1

1. List all ingredients in the recipe and their amounts.
2. Convert each ingredient into the number of exchanges it provides. Refer to the table on page 73.
3. Total each exchange group for the entire recipe.
4. Divide the total exchanges by the number of servings in the recipe. You can round off these numbers to the nearest one-half exchange. Anything less than one-half does not need to be counted. Figure 1 shows an example of a recipe that's been converted using this method.

Tuna Rice Casserole (Yield: 8 servings, 1 cup)

Ingredients	Starch	Fruit	Milk	Other Carb	Veg	Meat	Fat	Free
1 cup wild rice	6							
¼ cup chopped onion								free
¼ cup margarine							10	
¼ cup flour	1½							
1 cup chicken broth								free
1½ cups evaporated skim milk			3					
2 (6⅛ oz) cans tuna, water packed						12 lean		
¼ cup diced pimento								free
2 Tbsp parsley								free
½ tsp salt								free
½ tsp pepper								free
½ cup almonds, chopped						1½ med. fat	6½	
Total Exchanges	8½	0	3		0	13½	16½	
Total Exchanges ÷ Total Number of Servings	1	0	Trace		0	2	2	

1 cup tuna rice casserole = 1 starch, 2 lean meat, 2 fat or 1 starch, 2 med. fat meat, 1 fat

Figure 1. Recipe conversion using exchange method.

Method 2

1. List all ingredients in the recipe and their amounts.
2. List the amount of carbohydrate, protein, and fat in each ingredient. Refer to the table on page 73.
3. Total the grams of carbohydrate, the grams of protein, and the grams of fat for the entire recipe.
4. Divide the grams of carbohydrate, the grams of protein, and the grams of fat each by the number of servings in the recipe.
5. Follow the steps for converting the results to exchanges as shown in appendix 4. Figure 2 shows an example of a recipe that has been converted using this method.

Recipe Name: Sesame Cookies (Yield: 24 cookies)

Ingredients	Carbohydrate (grams)	Protein (grams)	Fat (grams)
2 Tbsp sesame seeds			
2 cups sifted flour	174	22	2
¼ tsp salt			
½ cup margarine			98
¼ cup shortening			56
1 cup sugar	199		
1 egg		6	6
1 tsp vanilla			
Total Nutrients	373	28	162
Total Nutrients ÷ Total Number of Servings	16	1	7
1 starch	15	3	
1 ½ fat			8

1 cookie = 1 other carbohydrate, 1½ fat or 1 carbohydrate choice, 1½ fat

Figure 2. Recipe conversion using grams of carbohydrate, protein, and fat.

Recipe Modifications and Substitutions

Ingredient	*Modification/Substitution*
Bacon, 2 strips	1 oz lean Canadian bacon or 1 oz lean ham
Bouillon cubes or granules	Low-sodium bouillon
Butter	Margarine
Cheese, regular	Reduced-fat or skim milk cheese
Chocolate, baking, 1 oz or 1 square	3 Tbsp cocoa + 1 Tbsp or less vegetable oil if needed
Cream cheese	Light cream cheese or 4 Tbsp margarine blended with 1 cup low-fat cottage cheese, salt to taste; small amount of skim milk is needed in blending
Cream, heavy, 1 cup	1 cup evaporated skim milk or 1 cup Poly Perx® or ⅔ cup skim milk and ⅓ cup oil
Cream, light	Equal portions of skim milk or 1% milk or evaporated skim milk
Egg, 1 whole	¼ cup egg substitute or 1 egg white +1 tsp vegetable oil or 2 egg whites, whipped
Evaporated milk	Evaporated skim milk
Fat in baked recipes	Use no more than 1 to 2 Tbsp of added oil or fat per cup of flour. Increase low-fat moist or liquid ingredients, such as buttermilk, to add moistness
½ to ⅓ cup oil in baking	Equal amount of applesauce or equal amount of baby-food fruits or 1 cup dried figs or dates pureed with ¾ cup water and 1 tsp vanilla
Flour, all-purpose, 1 cup	1 cup whole wheat flour minus 1 Tbsp oil called for in recipe, and increase liquid by 1 to 2 Tbsp, or ½ cup white + ½ cup whole wheat flour, or ¾ cup white + ¼ cup wheat germ or bran
Frosting	Sprinkle powdered sugar
Fruit, syrup-packed, canned	Fruit, juice-packed, canned
Garlic, onion, and celery salt	Garlic, onion, and celery powder

Ingredient	*Modification/Substitution*
Gelatin, regular	Sugar-free gelatin mix or fruit juice mixed with unflavored gelatin
Mayonnaise	Plain yogurt + 1 Tbsp mayonnaise per cup or reduced-calorie mayonnaise
Milk, whole	Skim milk or 1% milk
Rice, white	Brown rice
Oil	Vegetable oil spray to keep foods from sticking
Salad dressing	Nonfat or light salad dressing
Salt in recipes	Reduce amount or eliminate; use spices and herbs
Shortening or lard, 1 cup	¾ cup vegetable oil or ½ cup vegetable oil + ¼ cup other liquid
Shortening, ½ cup	⅓ cup vegetable oil
Soup, condensed	White sauce (1 cup skim milk + 2 Tbsp flour + 2 Tbsp margarine)
Cream of celery, 1 can	1 cup sauce + ¼ cup chopped celery
Cream of chicken, 1 can	1 cup sauce + chicken bouillon powder
Cream of mushroom, 1 can	1 cup sauce + 1 small can drained mushrooms
Sour cream, 1 cup	1 cup nonfat plain yogurt or 1 cup low-fat cottage cheese + 2 Tbsp lemon juice + 1 Tbsp skim milk or light sour cream
Sugar in baked recipes	Reduce amount by ½ to ⅓ of the original amount; use no more than ¼ cup added sweetener (sugar, honey, molasses) per cup of flour
Tuna or salmon, oil-packed	Water-packed tuna or salmon
Vegetables, canned with added salt	Fresh or frozen vegetables or low-salt canned or rinsed canned vegetables

Common Baking and Cooking Ingredients

Food	Serving	Carb. (grams)	Protein (grams)	Fat (grams)	Exchanges
Starches					
Biscuit mix	½ cup	37	4	8	2½ starch, 1 fat
Bread crumbs, dry	1 cup	65	11	4	4 starch
Graham cracker crumbs	1 cup	90	8	14	6 starch, 2 fat
Chow mein noodles	½ cup	17	3	8	1 starch, 1 fat
Cornmeal, uncooked	1 cup	117	11	5	7½ starch
Cornstarch	2 Tbsp	14	–	–	1 starch
Cream soup, undiluted	1 can (10¾ oz)	22	5	19	1½ starch, 3½ fat
Flour					
All-purpose	1 cup	87	11	1	6 starch
Cake, sifted	1 cup	79	8	1	5 starch
Rye	1 cup	66	10	2	4½ starch
Whole wheat	1 cup	80	16	2	5 starch
Macaroni					
Uncooked, 3½ oz	1 cup	79	7	trace	5 starch
Cooked	1 cup	41	7	1	3 starch
Noodles, egg					
Uncooked, 2½ oz	1 cup	59	7	1	4 starch
Cooked	1 cup	40	8	3	2½ starch
Oatmeal, uncooked	1 cup	54	15	6	3½ starch, 1 fat
Rice, white & brown					
Uncooked	¼ cup	39	3	–	2½ starch
Cooked	1 cup	36	3	1	2½ starch
Wild, uncooked	¼ cup	21	4	–	1½ starch
Long grain, instant, dry	¼ cup	26	2	–	2 starch
Long grain, instant cooked	1 cup	40	4	–	2½ starch
Spaghetti					
Uncooked, 3½ oz	1 cup	79	7	trace	5 starch
Cooked	1 cup	41	7	1	2½ starch

Food	Serving	Carb. (grams)	Protein (grams)	Fat (grams)	Exchanges
Wheat germ, 1 oz	¼ cup	13	9	3	1 starch, 1 lean meat
Dairy Products					
Butter or margarine	¼ cup	–	–	49	10 fat
	½ cup	–	–	98	20 fat
Cheese					
Cheddar, shredded	1 cup	2	29	37	4 high fat meat, 1 fat
Cream	4 oz	3	8	40	1 high fat meat, 6 fat
Mozzarella, part-skim, shredded	1 cup	3	28	18	4 med. fat meat
Parmesan, grated	¼ cup	1	8	6	1 med. fat meat
Cream					
Half and half	½ cup	5	3	14	3 fat
Sour	½ cup	4	3	20	5 fat
Heavy, not whipped	¼ cup	2	1	22	4 fat
Heavy, whipped	½ cup	2	1	22	4 fat
Egg					
Whole	1 medium	–	6	6	1 med. fat meat
Yolk	1 medium	–	3	5	1 fat
Milk					
Condensed, sweetened	⅓ cup	54	8	9	1 milk, 3 fruit
Evaporated, whole	½ cup	12	8	10	1 milk, 2 fat
Evaporated, skim	½ cup	14	9	–	1 milk
Nonfat dry, instant	1 cup	31	21	–	2½ milk
Yogurt					
Plain, nonfat	1 cup	17	12	–	1 milk
Fats, Oils, Chocolate, Cocoa					
Carob powder	1 cup	113	6	2	7½ starch
Chocolate chips	1 cup	105	8	48	7 other carb, 10 fat
Chocolate flavored syrup	2 Tbsp	17	1	1	1 other carb

Food	Serving	Carb. (grams)	Protein (grams)	Fat (grams)	Exchanges
Chocolate, bitter unsweetened	1 oz	7	4	16	½ other carb, 3 fat
Cocoa powder	¼ cup	16	6	2	1 starch
Mayonnaise	½ cup	1	1	88	17½ fat
Mayonnaise-type salad dressing	½ cup	14	1	55	1 starch, 11 fat
Olives, sliced	½ cup	2	1	15	3 fat
Shortening	½ cup	–	–	111	22 fat
Vegetable oil	½ cup	–	–	111	22 fat
Fruits and Vegetables					
Barbecue sauce	3 Tbsp	15	–	1	1 other carb
Catsup	½ cup	30	2	1	2 other carb
Chili sauce	½ cup	30	2	1	2 other carb
Dates	1 cup	130	4	1	8½ fruit
Raisins	½ cup	55	2	–	3½ fruit
Tomatoes or tomato juice	1 cup	9	2		2 veg
Tomato sauce or puree	1 cup	20	4	1	1 starch or 4 veg
Sugars and Syrups					
Corn syrup	1 cup	242	–	–	16 other carb
Gelatin powder, regular	3 oz box	74	6	–	5 other carb
Honey	1 cup	264	1	–	17½ other carb
Molasses					
Light	1 cup	213	–	–	14 other carb
Dark	1 cup	180	–	–	12 other carb
Sugar					
Brown, packed	1 cup	212	–	–	14 other carb
Powdered, sifted	1 cup	100	–	–	6½ other carb

Food	Serving	Carb. (grams)	Protein (grams)	Fat (grams)	Exchanges
Powdered, unsifted	1 cup	119	–	–	8 other carb
White	1 cup	199	–	–	13 other carb
Nuts					
Almonds	½ cup	15	14	41	1 starch, 1½ med. fat meat, 6½ fat
Cashews	1 cup	29	17	46	2 starch, 1½ med. fat meat, 7½ fat
Coconut, shredded	1 cup	33	2	24	2 fruit, 5 fat
Peanuts	1 oz (¼ cup)	5	7	14	1 med. fat meat, 2 fat
Peanut butter	1 cup	34	76	137	2 starch, 10 med. fat meat, 17 fat
Pecans	1 cup	13	9	73	1 starch, 1 med. fat meat, 13½ fat
Sunflower seed kernels	½ cup	14	17	34	1 starch, 2 med. fat meat, 5 fat
Walnuts	1 cup	16	15	64	1 starch, 2 med. fat meat, 10½ fat
Meats					
Chicken, canned	5½ oz	–	34	18	5 lean meat
Ground beef, lean	1 lb raw	–	79	66	11 med. fat meat, 2 fat
Salmon, pink, canned	16 oz can	–	93	27	13 lean meat
Tuna, canned					
water-packed	6⅛ oz can	–	44	3	6 lean meat
oil-packed	6½ oz can	–	45	30	6 med. fat meat

CHAPTER 8

Dining Out With Exchanges

Calorie for calorie, foods eaten away from home generally have more fat and fewer nutrients than foods eaten at home. However, a growing number of restaurants and delicatessens are actively promoting nutrition and low-calorie fare. Many have low-fat and low-sodium choices that are clearly indicated on the menu. In addition, almost three out of four restaurants report they will alter the way they prepare foods at a diner's request. This includes serving a sauce or salad dressing on the side, cooking without salt, cooking with margarine or vegetable oil instead of a saturated fat, and broiling or baking a food instead of frying it.

Sauces and cooking techniques can make the difference between low-fat cuisine and high-calorie, high-fat meals. Chicken, turkey, fish, or lean red meat can be the start of a healthy dish, but adding mayonnaise-based dressings, butter, or cream-based sauces or frying in oil will turn the final product into a high-fat choice.

How often you eat out also determines how careful you need to be in the selection of menu choices. If you eat more than five meals per week out, then your meals need to closely match your meal plan. If you eat out only once a month or on special occasions, you can take more liberties with your selections.

When dining away from home, bring your good common sense with you. You can follow your meal plan and enjoy yourself at the same time. For gastronomic adventures, follow these simple guidelines.

Guidelines for Smart Diners

Know your meal plan. Know how many exchanges or carbohydrate choices you are allowed for each meal and then make selections accordingly. Carrying a wallet-sized summary of your meal plan, which lists the exchanges or number of servings for the foods you routinely eat, can be a helpful reminder. You can generally determine which list a selection on the menu falls into. Use your choices wisely.

You also may decide ahead of time where you will eat and what you are going to order so that you are sure to choose something that fits into your meal plan. By doing this you won't be tempted by inappropriate food choices. Order first and be the trendsetter. Have you noticed how often the rest of the people at a table order what the first person chooses? By ordering first you won't be influenced by others. Instead they will probably follow your example, and all will benefit!

Watch portion sizes and learn to estimate a "serving." Don't feel you have to eat all the food served. If portion sizes are too large for your meal plan, share your entrée, leave the food, or ask for a doggie bag. You can save the extra food and have it for lunch the next day.

If the food is meat, fish, or poultry, then regardless of its exotic name, a one-ounce serving will equal one meat exchange. One-half cup of pasta, one-half cup of a starchy vegetable, or one ounce of a bread product (about the size of a medium-sized dinner roll) will equal one starch or one carbohydrate choice. One-half cup or the equivalent of a medium-sized fresh fruit is one fruit exchange.

Train your eyes to measure portion sizes. You can develop this ability at home by using measuring utensils to portion out various foods and learning to "eyeball" appropriate serving sizes. After you become a good judge of portion sizes, check your accuracy occasionally. It's easy for a teaspoon of margarine, a tablespoon of salad dressing, or a half-cup of mashed potatoes to become larger and larger over time.

Watch preparation. How foods are cooked affects their calorie and fat values. Choose foods that are broiled, roasted, steamed, poached, or stir-fried. Ask if fat is used in cooking the food, and if so what type. You must add one starch (one carbohydrate choice) and one to two fat exchanges per serving of a food that is breaded and fried, such as fried chicken or shrimp. The same food baked or broiled without breading would not carry the additional starch and fat exchanges. Also, meat weights listed on menus refer to the portion size before cooking. Meat loses about one quarter of its weight in cooking, so an eight-ounce steak is approximately six ounces or six meat exchanges when cooked.

How a food is served also can be a clue to making good choices. Think about what accompanies the selection such as gravy, sauce, sour cream, or whipped cream. All of these add fat and calories. Foods served with tomato or cocktail sauce, or in broth or wine, are nutrition winners. Avoid foods described as buttery, creamed, scalloped, or au gratin. Watch out for cream, butter, cheese, and hollandaise sauces as well. While you are learning how to use your meal plan, it may be wise to select foods that are prepared simply and to avoid rich sauces and casseroles with many ingredients.

Take charge and ask questions. If you are not sure how a dish is prepared, ask the person waiting on you. You should ask not only about how a certain item is prepared, but also about the portion size. Find out how many ounces of meat, fish, potatoes, or vegetables are in a standard portion.

Be assertive in requesting how you want your meal served; you are the one paying for it! For example, you can ask that your food not be buttered before broiling, that a sauce be omitted or served on the side so you can control the amount you eat, or that a high-fat cheese to be melted on top be omitted. Also, some restaurants now have low-sugar or light syrups, jams, and jellies and nonfat or light salad dressings. These items may not appear on the menu but may be available if you ask for them.

Plan ahead. You can move all the fat exchanges you can spare from another time of day to your meal out. It is a good idea to save as many fat exchanges as you can, because meals out usually contain more fat than meals at home. You might want to be careful of fat exchanges the next day as well. If you feel you have "blown it" and eaten too much, remember that you can exercise. Dancing, bicycling, or walking briskly can help you feel better and get back on track.

If you have diabetes. Meals eaten out or for social occasions often are served later than meals eaten at home. If you take insulin and a meal is delayed by one hour, have one carbohydrate choice (fifteen grams of carbohydrate) at the scheduled meal time. This is particularly important if the delay is unexpected and you have already taken your insulin injection at the usual time. If you are in a restaurant and your meal is delayed, ask your server for some crackers or a bread basket.

If your evening meal is delayed for longer than one and a half hours, you can eat your evening snack at your usual meal time, and eat the meal when it is served. You also can adjust your insulin regimen to accommodate changes in meal times. Talk to your health care provider about how to do this.

An important word of caution: If your bedtime blood glucose level is higher than usual after a large restaurant or special occasion meal, *do not* take extra insulin at that time. Taking extra insulin after the fact really doesn't help. By the time the insulin is at its peak of action, the elevated blood glucose from the meal will have decreased. The time to take extra insulin is *before* a larger-than-usual meal, not after. Also, you only need to take one or two extra units; taking more can cause more harm than good. Check with your health care provider on how to make adjustments in your insulin.

Understanding Restaurant Menu Terms

The name of a menu item or its description can help you recognize low-fat and high-fat preparation methods so you can make healthy selections. As always, though, portion size is key. Too much of any food can add calories you don't need. The following definitions will help you find healthy items on any menu.

A la Grecque: Usually cooked in oil and vinegar or lemon juice with seasonings; this is a good choice

A la King: A white sauce with mushrooms and pimiento or green pepper

Au Gratin: Cooking process that produces a crisp, golden brown crust, usually formed by baking or broiling bread crumbs, cheese, and butter; or dishes that will crust on their own accord

Au Jus: Meat served in its own juice

Au Maigre: With no meat, which means less fat

Béarnaise: Rich sauce made with egg yolks, tarragon, butter, shallots, vinegar, and sometimes white wine

Bordelaise: Brown sauce seasoned with wine and shallots, garnished with poached marrow and parsley

Cacciatore: Tomato sauce with mushrooms, herbs, and other seasonings; a good choice

Chasseur (Hunter's Sauce): Brown sauce with tomatoes, mushrooms, herbs, and other seasonings; this is a good choice

Coq au Vin: Sautéed in red wine and brown sauce with mushrooms and onions

Creole: Spicy combination of tomatoes, green peppers, okra, onions, and seasonings, usually cooked in oil; this is a good choice if oil is kept to a minimum

Deviled: Prepared with hot or savory seasoning usually after being finely chopped; this is a good choice

Hollandaise: Usually made with egg yolks, butter, lemon juice, or vinegar

Jambalaya: Spicy dish of rice, tomatoes, onions, peppers, and other seasonings; usually includes sausage; without the sausage, this is a good choice

Julienne: Cut into match-like strips

Kiev: Stuffed with seasoned butter and flour; often deep-fried in oil

Kippered: Lightly salted and smoked

Lyonnaise: Cooked with pieces of onion and butter

Marinara: Tomato-based sauce with onion, garlic, and seasonings; this is a good choice for pasta

Mornay: A béchamel sauce with cream and grated cheese, sometimes egg yolks

Parmigiana: Covered with bread crumbs and Parmesan cheese, then sautéed in butter and served with tomato sauce; usually includes mozzarella cheese as well

Remoulade: Chopped pickles and capers with mayonnaise, tarragon, and spices

Scalloppine: Meat pounded very thin, floured, and broiled or sautéed in wine sauce; this is a good choice if little or no oil is used in cooking

Thermidor: Cream sauce seasoned with wine and herbs or mustard

Good Choices When Dining Out

Appetizers
Tomato juice
Vegetable juice
Fruit juice
Broth-based soup
Tomato-based soup
Bouillon
Consommé
Vegetable platter
Fruit cocktail
Shrimp cocktail
Crab cocktail

Salads
Green salad
Fresh fruit salad

Dressings
Lemon wedge
Oil and vinegar
Low-fat dressing
Reduced-fat dressing

Salad Bars
Load up:
Raw vegetables

Sparingly:
Cheese
Olives
Seeds
Croutons
Hard-boiled eggs
Bacon

Skip:
Potato salad
Pasta salad
Coleslaw

Breads
Dinner roll
French bread
Pita bread
Rye
Pumpernickel
Sourdough bread
Plain muffin
Crackers
Popover
Bread sticks
Melba toast
Ry-Krisp
Bagel
English muffin

Entrées

Meat/Fish/Poultry (roasted, baked, broiled, blackened, grilled, stir-fried, or barbecued)

Filet mignon

Shish kebob

Steamed clams

Softshell crab

Steamed crab

Broiled or steamed lobster

Grilled scallops

Mussels

Venison

Leg of lamb

Chicken teriyaki

Beef teriyaki

Chicken fajitas

Beef fajitas

Chili

Pasta with tomato sauce

Grilled sandwich

Pita sandwich

Soup (meat, vegetable, legume)

Side Dishes

Mashed potatoes

Baked potatoes

Steamed potatoes

Rice

Rice pilaf

Noodles

Pasta

Corn on the cob

Raw vegetables

Stewed vegetables

Steamed vegetables

Boiled vegetables

Grilled vegetables

Roasted vegetables

Stir-fried vegetables

Desserts

Fresh fruit

Frozen nonfat yogurt

Plain ice cream

Sherbet

Fresh fruit sorbet

Sponge cake

Angel food cake

Cookie

See chapters 19 to 23 for ethnic choices and chapter 24 for fast-food selections.

If Alcohol Is Used

For many people alcoholic beverages have become an accepted part of social life. The decision to drink or not drink alcoholic beverages must be made by each individual. To make this decision, you need to be aware of the effects of alcohol on the body.

Alcohol is broken down in the liver by specific enzymes, but the liver can process less than one ounce of alcohol (about one drink) in an hour. When more than that amount enters the liver, it moves through the liver into the general blood circulation. When this happens, alcohol reaches the central nervous system and the brain, and the effects of alcohol on behavior begin. Initially it lifts the barriers of self-control, but alcohol is a depressant and it will eventually slow down brain activity. When the liver can handle the alcohol it will be metabolized or broken down.

Alcohol is a concentrated source of calories, yielding seven calories per gram. It provides energy but no other essential nutrients. An ounce and a half of 80 proof liquor contributes 100 calories. Beer and sweet wines contain carbohydrate as well as alcohol, so they have additional calories. If the calories from alcohol are not used as an immediate energy source, they are converted to fat and triglycerides. This is why too much alcohol can lead to a fatty liver, high blood fats (triglycerides), and weight gain.

Alcohol can be included in your meal plan if it is done wisely and you remember to count it. The following table gives nutrition and exchange values for various alcoholic beverages.

Composition of Alcoholic Beverages

Beverage	Serving	Alcohol (grams)	Carbohydrate (grams)	Calories	Exchanges
Beer					
Regular	12 oz	13	13	150	1 starch, 2 fat
Light	12 oz	11	5	100	2 fat
Non-alcoholic	12 oz	1.5	12	60–75	1 starch
Distilled Spirits					
Gin, rum, vodka, whiskey, scotch	1 ½ oz	14	trace	100	2 fat
Brandy, cognac	1 oz	11	trace	75	1 ½ fat

Beverage	Serving	Alcohol (grams)	Carbohydrate (grams)	Calories	Exchanges
Wines					
Dry white	5 oz	14	trace	110	2 fat
Red or rose	5 oz	14	trace	110	2 fat
Light	5 oz	7–12	1	65	1 fat
Wine cooler	12 oz	10–17	30	220	2 fruit, 2 fat
Sparkling Wines					
Champagne	4 oz	12	4	100	2 fat
Kosher	4 oz	12	12	132	1 starch, 2 fat
Dessert Wines					
Sherry	3 oz	14	2	125	2 fat
Sweet sherry, port, muscatel	3 oz	14	9	150	½ starch, 2 fat
Cordials, liqueurs	½ oz	13	18	160	1 starch, 2 fat
Cocktails					
Bloody Mary	5 oz	14	5	116	1 veg, 2 fat
Daiquiri	2 oz	14	2	111	2 fat
Manhattan	2 oz	17	2	178	2½ fat
Martini	2½ oz	22	trace	156	3½ fat
Old-fashioned	4 oz	26	trace	180	4 fat
Tom Collins	7½ oz	16	3	120	2½ fat
Mixes					
Mineral water	any	–	0	0	free
Sugar-free tonic	any	–	0	0	free
Club soda	any	–	0	0	free
Diet soda	any	–	0	0	free
Tomato juice	½ cup	–	5	25	1 veg
Bloody Mary mix	½ cup	–	5	25	1 veg
Fruit juice	½ cup	–	15	60	1 fruit

Diabetes and Alcohol

The metabolism of alcohol does not require insulin. In fact, alcohol increases the effect of insulin. Alcohol does not stimulate the pancreas to release insulin, but it enhances the glucose-lowering action of insulin or other glucose-lowering agents.

Well-controlled blood glucose levels are not affected by the moderate use of alcohol when it is consumed shortly before, during, or immediately after eating. However, if food is not eaten, alcohol can cause blood glucose levels to become dangerously low. Hypoglycemia can occur even before a person is aware of being mildly intoxicated. Two ounces of alcohol (one to two drinks) on an empty stomach is enough to produce hypoglycemia. People in poor control of their diabetes or who have exercised strenuously just before drinking alcohol usually have depleted carbohydrate stores and so are at special risk for hypoglycemia.

Occasionally, alcohol can cause blood glucose levels to become elevated, especially if alcohol intake is excessive. However, this is usually temporary and can be followed several hours later by a drop in blood glucose to below-normal levels.

Many people with diabetes can include alcohol with their meal plan by following some simple guidelines. These guidelines refer to occasional use of alcoholic beverages, which is defined as about two drinks not more than once or twice a week. If alcohol is used daily, the amount must be limited and the calories counted in your meal plan.

Drink alcohol only if your diabetes is in good control. Your health care provider can advise you on how to balance your food intake, exercise, and medication to achieve blood glucose control, and he or she will tell you if there is some reason you should avoid alcoholic beverages.

Drink alcohol in moderation. Sip slowly and make a drink last a long time. It's important also to always eat something when you have an alcoholic drink. Since symptoms of alcohol intoxication and hypoglycemia are similar, it is easy for other people to mistake a low blood sugar for intoxication and delay necessary treatment.

Limit yourself to no more than two of the following drinks each day. Each contains about the same amount of alcohol.

• 1.5 ounces of distilled spirits (hard liquor such as whiskey, scotch, rye, vodka, gin, cognac, rum, dry brandy)

- 4–5 ounces of wine
- 2 ounces of sherry
- 12 ounces of beer, preferably light

Count alcohol in your meal plan. For people of normal weight who take injected insulin, two of the above drinks can be used as an "extra." People with type II diabetes for whom weight is a concern must count the calories from alcohol in their meal plan. Calories are best substituted for fat exchanges because alcohol is metabolized in a manner similar to fat (each of the above amounts is equal to two fat exchanges). Avoid or limit alcohol consumption if you need to shed excess pounds. Since alcohol provides calories, most of which your body stores as fat, and no other nutrients, losing weight may become more difficult when you drink, even occasionally.

Avoid sweet liqueurs and cordials, which can have a sugar content as high as fifty percent. Beer and ale contain malt sugar and need to be counted in the meal plan. Light beer is recommended because it has about three to six grams of carbohydrate in a twelve-ounce can, while regular beer has thirteen to eighteen grams of carbohydrate per can.

Don't let a drink make you careless. Alcohol can have a relaxing effect and may dull judgment. Be sure meals and snacks are taken on time and selected with care. Too much alcohol may lead to further dietary indiscretion. Avoid hypoglycemia (low blood sugar) the morning after drinking alcohol by setting your alarm before you retire to help you get up, then test your blood glucose and eat your usual breakfast.

Carry identification. Visible identification should be carried or worn when drinking away from home. An insulin reaction can appear too much like intoxication to take any chances.

Alcohol should be avoided if you have:

- a history of alcohol abuse;
- elevated triglyceride levels, gastritis, or pancreatitis;
- kidney or heart disease;
- frequent hypoglycemic reactions;
- gestational diabetes; or
- diabetes and are pregnant.

Alcohol also interacts with barbiturates and tranquilizers, sleeping pills, antihistamines, cold remedies, and a number of other drugs.

In Summary

When dining away from home, it's helpful to do some planning. Plan where you will eat, what you will eat, and how much you will eat.

Where: It helps if you're familiar with the menu of the restaurant. The more choices on the menu, the more apt you are to find choices appropriate for you.

What: Familiarity with your meal plan is of primary importance. Know what exchanges you can use for the meal you are eating away from home. If you drink alcohol, do it wisely and count it in your meal plan.

How much: Judging portion sizes by "eyeballing" them will help you decide how much to take home and save for another meal.

By planning, understanding your meal plan, and correctly judging portion sizes, you can enjoy dining away from home.

CHAPTER 9

Travel and Meal Planning

Planning is essential before taking any trip—a one-day excursion, a weekend camping trip, or an international trek—and meal planning needs the same consideration that travel arrangements and sleeping accommodations do. When you are following a meal plan for weight loss or a chronic health condition, you need to take vacation or business travel in stride and not allow it to interfere with healthy eating. By thinking ahead and being prepared you can travel, enjoy exotic foods, and have fun, all the while following your meal plan.

Travel schedules, whether you go by airplane, car, bus, or train, are frequently upset. Delays are common. Have some healthy, non-perishable foods with you in your pocket, purse, car, or flight bag. They can be used as snacks when meals are delayed, when driving for extended periods, or as fuel for increased physical activity. This is especially important for people who have diabetes. The following list gives some options for quick snacks.

Food	Quantity	Carbohydrate Choices	Exchanges
Chips or snack foods	¾–1 oz	1	1 starch, 1–2 fat
Crackers	4 or 5 (1 oz)	1	1 starch, 0–1 fat
Dried fruit	¼ cup (½ oz)	1	1 fruit
Fruit juice	4 oz	1	1 fruit
Fruit rolls or bars	1 (½ oz)	1	1 fruit
Granola bar	1	1	1 starch, 1 fat
Nuts, sunflower seeds	1 oz	0	1 med. fat meat, 2 fat
Pretzels	¾ oz	1	1 starch

When traveling, it can get tiresome (and expensive!) eating all your meals in restaurants. It is quite easy and often healthier to prepare some of your own meals, especially breakfast and lunch, from foods purchased in a supermarket. Breakfasts can be prepared in your hotel room from canned fruit juice or fresh fruit; dry cereal; a bagel, bread, or hard roll; milk; and a beverage. There are many travel appliances that allow you to heat water for instant beverages or hot cereal. Small travel coffee makers also are widely available, and you can take along a thermos for milk. For lunch you may enjoy a picnic. Try lean meat and low-fat cheese, buns, and fruit. Put them together and you have a healthy, inexpensive meal with little or no waste.

Air Travel

Airline food is not known as being terribly healthy, so it is important to plan ahead when traveling by air. When you book your flight, you can order a special meal through your travel agent or the airline. You must make your request at least forty-eight hours ahead of departure. The low-fat or vegetarian meal is appropriate for most meal plans. If you have diabetes, tell the flight attendant, mention that you have ordered a special meal, and stress that it is important to have your meals served on time.

Sometimes the special meal doesn't arrive, even if you have ordered it well in advance. If it doesn't, take the regular meal. You can choose foods from it and substitute other things from a food supply that you carry with you. It's a good idea to carry convenient and healthy snacks like fruit with you for these occasions, and also for times when flights are delayed or canceled. Also, be sure to drink plenty of liquids before and while traveling by air. Drink one cup of a nonalcoholic liquid for each hour you are in the air.

The need to carry snacks is vitally important if you have diabetes. Many airlines do not offer full food service, and you can easily get caught without the food you need to stay on your schedule. Always carry snacks with you when you travel.

International Travel

No matter where you travel, food is made of carbohydrate, protein, and fat. A leafy vegetable grown in Japan is still a vegetable exchange. A small to medium fruit still counts as a fruit exchange. Starches or grains are starch exchanges; meat, fish, cheese, and eggs are meat exchanges. And oil is a fat exchange, whether it's sesame oil or whale oil. But when you are faced with unfamiliar foods and terminology in a foreign land, it may be difficult to know how to fit foods into your meal plan. One common difference in foreign countries is the use of "joules" instead of "calories"; four joules equal one calorie.

Chapters 19 through 23 discuss eating customs in different countries and list exchanges and carbohydrate choices for many ethnic foods that you might want to try, either here or abroad. Look for foods you want to try and then look for the exchange information in the appropriate chapters in this book. This will help you think ahead so you can enjoy the experience of trying different meals on your trip. If you can't find what you're looking for, go to the library or bookstore for guides to eating out in the region you are traveling to.

The chart below is a general guide to portion sizes and exchanges for unfamiliar foods that you can't find specific information about. As long as you know what type of food it is—starch, fruit, milk, etc.—you can follow the guidelines given to know how much to eat and how to count it in your meal plan.

Exchange List	Universal Portion	Carbohydrate Choices	Exchanges
Starch	½ cup	1	1 starch
Fruit	½ cup	1	1 fruit
Milk	1 cup	1	1 milk
Vegetable	½ cup	0	1 veg
Meat	1 oz	0	1 meat
Fat	1 tsp	0	1 fat
Combination (casserole)	1 cup	2	2 starch, 2 meat, 1–2 fat

Soup, in particular, is a common and healthy food often eaten as a light lunch or dinner appetizer when dining away from home. As a general rule, one cup of a broth-type soup (noodles, vegetables, rice) is counted as one starch exchange; one cup of a cream or bean soup is one starch and one fat exchange. A *bowl* of any kind of soup is two starch and one to two fats.

The water in foreign countries, including ice cubes, often is not safe to drink, and milk may not be pasteurized. Tea or coffee can be three-fourths cream or milk. Good beverage options in these situations include plain coffee or tea, bottled mineral water, wine in moderation, and fruit juice. Sugar-free soft drinks are becoming more available around the world, but they are still hard to find in some countries. Many so-called "diabetic" drinks are sweetened with either fructose or sorbitol, which have as many calories as sugar. It's better to stick with bottled mineral water.

Food preparation is not always checked or regulated by foreign countries, and precautions are necessary in order to avoid getting sick. This is especially true in South and Central America, Asia, Africa, and Mexico. Milk products such as ice cream and cream sauces; raw or rare meats, poultry, and fish; soft cheeses; fresh fruit with skin; raw vegetables; foods displayed or sold in open markets; and poorly refrigerated foods are all potential sources of organisms that can cause traveler's diarrhea and other illnesses. Be sure to seek treatment at the first sign of diarrhea, which can quickly become serious if not attended to.

Guidelines for Diabetes

Taking appropriate precautions and planning your trip with your diabetes in mind can make travel safer and more enjoyable. Unfortunately, some people feel they would like to take a vacation from their diabetes when they are away from home. This can cause serious problems. You need to continue monitoring your blood glucose and following your meal plan so you can avoid insulin reactions and the chance of ketoacidosis. With planning you can fully enjoy your time away.

Traveling with insulin. If you take insulin, carry it with you along with syringes, blood glucose monitoring equipment, and urine ketone testing materials. Bring extra regular insulin along to use in case you become ill. Pack these necessities in a carry-on bag instead of a checked-through suitcase, in case your luggage is delayed or lost. You don't want to spend precious travel time trying to find glucose strips, insulin, or syringes.

If you plan to be gone for a long time, you may want to contact your insulin manufacturer to make sure insulin is available in the country you will be visiting. A foreign country may carry the insulin you use, but it may have a different name. U-100 insulin and U-100 syringes are not available in all countries. The key is to use the same type of syringe as your insulin. If U-40 insulin is all that's available, you also must use a U-40 syringe.

Protect your strips and insulin from extremes in temperature—temperatures above 86 degrees Fahrenheit or below freezing may produce inaccurate results. You can keep your insulin in a plastic bag in a wide-mouthed thermos jug lined with a wet washcloth. This way, the insulin stays cool and the vials won't break.

A well-equipped medical kit containing bandages, antiseptic solution, a decongestant, motion sickness pills, and sunscreen also is invaluable to the traveler.

Changing time zones. If you take insulin, it is sometimes necessary to make adjustments in your dose or schedule to accommodate time changes. When traveling in the United States and the time change is only one, two, or three hours, you can gradually change your morning insulin injection time. Each morning move it one-half hour ahead or behind—depending on which direction you are going—until you are back on schedule. However, if you plan to jet across several time zones, such as to Europe or Asia, you will need to make adjustments in your insulin dose and injection time. The following are general guidelines for adjusting insulin during travel. Be sure to talk to your health care provider for individual advice.

When you lose four or more hours from your day, such as when traveling east from the United States to Europe, you may need to decrease your intermediate-acting insulin dose. On the day you travel, decrease your morning dose for morning travel, or decrease your evening dose for travel later in the day. Decrease the dose by whatever percentage of twenty-four hours you will lose. For example, if the time difference is six hours, you would decrease the intermediate-acting insulin by twenty-five percent, because six hours is twenty-five percent of twenty-four hours. Once you arrive at your destination, you can go back to your usual insulin regimen.

When gaining four or more hours in your day, such as when traveling west from Europe to the United States, you may need to increase your regular insulin dose or add an injection of regular insulin to cover the additional time. Take your usual morning dose, then take extra units of regular or an additional injection of regular before the second in-flight meal. Ten percent of your total twenty-four-hour dose is a good starting point for adjustments. For example, if your total daily amount of regular and intermediate-acting insulin is forty units, you would add four units of regular insulin. Once you arrive at your destination, you can go back to your usual insulin regimen.

Insulin regimens using Humalog® (a very rapid-acting insulin) with an intermediate-acting insulin (background insulin) give you the most flexibility. However, you still may need to increase or decrease your dose of background insulin to accommodate the gain or loss of time when traveling. Humalog® should always be taken at the time of the meal, not thirty minutes before the meal, as with regular insulin.

Changing meal times. Airplane travel is not the only time your eating schedule may be disrupted. In many foreign countries, it is customary to eat late evening meals. In this case, you would have your evening snack at the usual evening meal time, and eat your dinner at the later hour. In Latin countries (Spain, Portugal, and South America), lunch often is served at 2 p.m. and dinner at 10 p.m. To adjust your meal plan accordingly, begin by having a substantial breakfast. Depending on the amount of exercise and activity planned, you also may need a late morning snack between 11 a.m. and noon. You may move your usual afternoon snack to this late morning time. You can then eat lunch at 2 p.m., have an early evening snack around 6 p.m., and eat dinner at 10 p.m.

Part of the fun of foreign travel is experiencing a different culture, and food is a big part of any culture. With planning and a few changes in your schedule, you can participate fully and enjoy new experiences. There are also more flexible insulins and regimens available today which can help you handle travel and meal-time changes more easily. Ask your health care provider about these possibilities.

Changes in activities. When traveling, you are likely to do a great deal of walking and sightseeing. If this is different from your usual activity pattern, you may need changes in your food intake and insulin.

If you increase your activity level, it is important to include extra carbohydrate snacks. For moderate exercise, start with an additional fruit or starch serving (one carbohydrate choice, or fifteen grams of carbohydrate). For more strenuous activity of a longer duration you may also need to decrease your insulin dose. If you have any questions contact your health care provider ahead of time.

Other precautions. Always carry a source of glucose with you so you can treat hypoglycemia (too low of a blood glucose level) immediately. Also, your travel partner should know how to give you glucagon. Glucagon can be used to treat hypoglycemia in a semiconscious or unconscious person, or when a person refuses or is unable to take food or drink by mouth. Glucagon, like insulin, must be given by injection. Glucagon is now available in a pre-filled syringe, but someone with you must know how to give it to you correctly.

It is not unusual to become ill while traveling. Nausea, vomiting, and diarrhea can occur, especially when traveling to foreign countries. If you become ill, it is essential to test your blood glucose a minimum of four times a day (before meals and the evening snack) and to check your urine for ketones. If your blood glucose levels are above 240 mg/dl and urine tests show moderate to large ketones, call a doctor. You may have an infection that needs to be treated.

You need to take additional insulin when you are sick and have high blood glucose levels and moderate to large ketones. A general guideline is to take an additional ten percent of your total insulin dose in the form of regular insulin every four to six hours. Take the extra insulin in addition to your usual insulin dose.

When traveling, carry spare prescriptions for prescription drugs and an explanatory letter from your physician regarding insulin syringes for customs officials. If needed, carry index cards with emergency phrases in the appropriate language (see appendix 5). If possible, have the name of an English-speaking physician in each city where you will be traveling (see appendix 1).

Always carry a card in your wallet and wear a wristband or necklace bearing medical identification. Travel companions should be aware that you have diabetes and should know what to do in case of an emergency such as hypoglycemia or hyperglycemia.

Medical Assistance for Travelers

If you should need a doctor abroad, the International Association for Medical Assistance to Travelers (IAMAT), a nonprofit organization, has set up centers in 125 countries with English- or French-speaking physicians who are on call at all hours of the day. IAMAT publishes an annual directory of medical centers, along with the names and addresses of associated physicians who have agreed to a set payment schedule for IAMAT cardholders. They also have information on climate, food, and sanitary conditions in countries you may be planning to visit. For more information, write to the IAMAT, 417 Center Street, Lewiston, New York 14092 (716-754-4883).

When traveling abroad, U.S. consuls are available to help you with serious medical, financial, and legal difficulties. Among their many services, U.S. embassies and consulates can:

- help you find medical assistance and inform your family and friends if you are ill or injured;

- assist you in replacing a lost passport or visa;

- arrange to have emergency funds sent by your family, friends, bank, or employer; and

- give you information on travel advisories, supply lists of local attorneys, and notarize documents.

In Summary

Remember, your meal plan travels with you. If you anticipate travel situations and plan carefully, you can follow your meal plan in any state, country, city, or wilderness area you visit.

PART THREE

Carbohydrate Exchange Lists

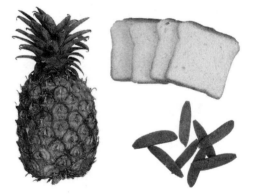

CHAPTER 10

Starch List

The Starch List includes a wide variety of foods—breads, cereals, rice, pasta, and other foods made from grains, as well as peas, beans, and lentils. Many of the foods on this list are good choices for you. Like all carbohydrate foods, starches give us energy, and they are often good sources of fiber as well. This list is discussed first because the foods on it are the foundation of a healthy meal plan. Depending on your caloric intake, plan to eat six to eleven starch servings each day.

Although most of the foods on the Starch List fit easily into a healthy diet, you can still make wise and not-so-wise choices. Choose foods that are high in fiber, such as whole grain breads, bran cereals, and dried peas, beans, and lentils. Foods that are the least "processed" are usually the highest in fiber. Eat fewer foods with added fat, such as potato chips and french fries.

Because foods on the Starch List will be frequent visitors at your table, be creative as you cook with them. Even foods that at first seem like bland basics may be more interesting and varied than you think. The many varieties of rice, for instance, have subtle differences in flavor and texture that can truly change the character of a dish. For example, basmati rice can lend an fragrant, authentic flavor to Indian and Asian dishes, while wild rice can add a hearty texture to soups and casseroles. Pastas have similar nuances—delicate angel hair is perfect for light pasta sauces, while larger noodles like mostaccioli and penne can balance fuller-bodied, spicy sauces. Pastas and breads flavored with spices, herbs, and vegetables can be found in almost any supermarket. Be adventurous in your selections!

Tips for Portion Sizes

- Bread or bread products: One exchange equals one ounce. To determine whether a hamburger or hot dog bun is one or two ounces, look at the total weight of the package and divide by the number of buns.

- Cereal, rice, or grain: One exchange usually equals one-third to one-half cup after cooking.

- Pasta: One exchange equals two ounces before cooking. For macaroni, rotini, and other small pastas, measure out one-half cup. For spaghetti, linguine, or other long pasta, two ounces held in a fist make a circle exactly the size of a U.S. penny.

- Soup is most easily counted as a starch in your meal plan. One cup of broth-based soup such as chicken noodle or vegetable beef is one starch exchange; a bowl is usually closer to two cups and would be counted as two starches. A cup of cream soup is one starch and one fat exchange.

One starch serving has:

15 grams carbohydrate

3 grams protein

½–1 gram fat

80 calories

One starch serving is:

1 ounce of a bread or snack product

¾ cup dry, unsweetened cereal

½ cup cooked cereal

4–5 snack crackers

½ cup pasta or starchy vegetable

⅓ cup rice, grains, stuffings

1 cup soup

½ cup cooked beans, peas, lentils

3 cups popcorn without added fat

STARCH LIST

Food	Quantity	Carbohydrate Choices	Exchanges
Bagel			
Medium (1 oz)	½ bagel	1	1 starch
Large (3.5 oz)	1 bagel	3½	3½ starch
Barley, cooked	⅓ cup	1	1 starch
Beans, baked			
Canned	⅓ cup	1	1 starch
	1 cup	3	3 starch, 1 very lean meat
Canned with franks	½ cup	1	1 starch, 1 high fat meat
Pork and beans	⅓ cup	1	1 starch
Beans, dried, cooked or canned	½ cup	1	1 starch, 1 very lean meat
	1 cup	2	2 starch, 1 very lean meat
Black beans	⅓ cup	1	1 starch
Garbanzo beans	⅓ cup	1	1 starch
Lima beans	½ cup	1	1 starch
Mung beans	⅓ cup	1	1 starch
Navy beans	⅓ cup	1	1 starch
Pinto beans	⅓ cup	1	1 starch
Beans, refried	⅓ cup	1	1 starch, 1 fat
Bean dip, canned	¼ cup	1	1 starch
Biscuit, baking soda or buttermilk	1 (2½" across)	1	1 starch, 1 fat
Black-eyed peas, canned	½ cup	1	1 starch
Bread; *see also* Pocket/Pita bread			
Boston brown bread	1 slice (3" across x ½" thick)	1	1 starch
Corn bread	2" square	1	1 starch, 1 fat
French bread	1 slice (3" thick)	1	1 starch
Home-baked or unsliced bread	1 oz	1	1 starch
Party bread (pumpernickel, rye)	4 slices	1	1 starch
Pumpernickel	1 slice	1	1 starch
Raisin bread, unfrosted	1 slice (1 oz)	1	1 starch

Food	Quantity	Carbohydrate Choices	Exchanges
Rye bread	1 slice	1	1 starch
Spoon bread	3½ oz	1	1 starch, 2 fat
White bread	1 slice (1 oz)	1	1 starch
Wheat bread	1 slice (1 oz)	1	1 starch
Bread, reduced calorie	2 slices (1½ oz)	1	1 starch
Bread, tea			
Banana bread	1 slice (1⁄16 loaf)	1	1 starch, 1 fat
Cranberry bread	1 slice (1½ oz)	1½	1½ starch, 1 fat
Pumpkin bread	1 slice (1½ oz)	1½	1½ starch, 1 fat
Bread crumbs, dry	3 Tbsp	1	1 starch
Breadsticks			
4" long x ½" thick	2 breadsticks	1	1 starch
4" long x ¼" thick	6 breadsticks	1	1 starch
Bulgur, cooked	½ cup	1	1 starch
Bun, hamburger or hot dog	1 bun (2 oz)	2	2 starch
Carob flour	2 Tbsp	1	1 starch
Cereal, ready-to-eat			
All Bran®	½ cup	1	1 starch
All Bran with Extra Fiber®	1 cup	1	1 starch
Apple Raisin Crisp®	⅔ cup	2	2 starch
Bran Buds®	½ cup	1	1 starch
Bran Chex®	½ cup	1	1 starch
Bran Flakes®	⅔ cup	1	1 starch
100% Bran®	½ cup	1	1 starch
Cheerios®	1 cup	1	1 starch
Cheerios®, Apple Cinnamon	½ cup	1	1 starch
Cheerios®, Honey Nut	½ cup	1	1 starch
Corn Bran®	½ cup	1	1 starch
Corn Chex®	¾ cup	1	1 starch
Corn Flakes®	¾ cup	1	1 starch
Crispy Wheaties 'n Raisins®	¾ cup	1½	1½ starch
Fiber One®	⅔ cup	1	1 starch
Fruit and Fibre®	½ cup	1	1 starch
Fruit Muesli®, all varieties	½ cup	2	2 starch

Food	Quantity	Carbohydrate Choices	Exchanges
Granola	¼ cup	1	1 starch, 1 fat
Granola, low-fat	¼ cup	1	1 starch
Grape Nuts®	¼ cup	1	1 starch
Grape Nuts® Flakes	¾ cup	1	1 starch
Kix®	1 cup	1	1 starch
Life®	⅔ cup	1	1 starch
Muesli®	¼ cup	1	1 starch
Mueslix® Crispy Blend	⅓ cup	1	1 starch
Mueslix® Golden Crunch	½ cup	1½	1½ starch
Nutri-Grain® Almond Raisin	⅔ cup	2	2 starch
Nutri-Grain® Raisin Bran	⅔ cup	1	1 starch
Nutri-Grain® Wheat	½ cup	1	1 starch
Oat bran	½ cup	1	1 starch
Oatmeal Crisp®	¾ cup	1	1 starch
Puffed Rice®	1½ cup	1	1 starch
Puffed Wheat®	1½ cup	1	1 starch
Raisin Bran®	½ cup	1	1 starch
Raisin Oat Bran®	¾ cup	2	2 starch
Rice Chex®	¾ cup	1	1 starch
Rice Krispies®	¾ cup	1	1 starch
Sunflakes Multi Grain®	¾ cup	1	1 starch
Shredded Wheat®	1 biscuit	1	1 starch
Shredded Wheat Squares®	½ cup	1	1 starch
Special K®	¾ cup	1	1 starch
Sugar-Frosted Flakes®	½ cup	1	1 starch
Team Flakes®	¾ cup	1	1 starch
Total®	¾ cup	1	1 starch
Total® Raisin Bran	1 cup	2	2 starch
Wheat Chex®	½ cup	1	1 starch
Wheaties®	¾ cup	1	1 starch
Cereal, hot			
Cream of Rice®	½ cup	1	1 starch
Cream of Wheat®	½ cup	1	1 starch
Farina	¾ cup	1	1 starch
Malt-O-Meal®	⅔ cup	1	1 starch

Food	Quantity	Carbohydrate Choices	Exchanges
Maypo®	½ cup	1	1 starch
Oat bran, cooked	⅓ cup	1	1 starch
Oatmeal, quick or Old Fashioned	½ cup	1	1 starch
Oatmeal, instant	1 pkt	1	1 starch
Oatmeal, instant flavored	1 pkt	2	2 starch
Ralston®	⅔ cup	1	1 starch
Roman Meal®	½ cup	1	1 starch
Wheatena®	½ cup	1	1 starch
Chapati, 5–6" across	1 chapati	1	1 starch
Cheese sauce (prepared with milk)	½ cup	1	1 starch, 1 high fat meat
Chestnuts	4 large or 6 small	1	1 starch
Corn			
Canned	½ cup	1	1 starch
Cob	1 medium ear	1	1 starch
Cream style	⅓ cup	1	1 starch
Pudding	½ cup	1	1 starch, 1 fat
Corn pone	1 cake (1½ oz)	1	1 starch, ½ fat
Cornmeal, dry	3 Tbsp	1	1 starch
Cornstarch	2 Tbsp	1	1 starch
Couscous, cooked	⅓ cup	1	1 starch
Cowpeas, frozen, boiled	½ cup	1	1 starch
Crackers			
Animal crackers	8 crackers	1	1 starch
American Classic®, all varieties	8 crackers	1	1 starch, 1 fat
Cheese-filled crackers	6 (1½ oz)	1½	1½ starch, 2 fat
Cheese Nips®	20 crackers	1	1 starch, 1 fat
Club®	8 crackers	1	1 starch, 1 fat
Goldfish crackers, all varieties	45 crackers	1	1 starch, 1 fat
Graham crackers, 2½" square	3 crackers	1	1 starch
Harvest Crisp®, all varieties	12 crackers	1	1 starch, 1 fat
Matzo, 6" across	1 wafer	1	1 starch
Matzo crackers, 1½" square	7 crackers	1	1 starch
Melba toast, long	4 slices	1	1 starch

Food	Quantity	Carbohydrate Choices	Exchanges
Melba toast, rounds	8 crackers	1	1 starch
Oat Bran Krisp®	4 triple crackers	1	1 starch, 1 fat
Oyster crackers	24 large or 42 small	1	1 starch
Peanut-butter filled crackers	6 (1½ oz)	1½	1½ starch, 2 fat
Ritz®, Hi Ho®	6 crackers	1	1 starch, 1 fat
Rusk	2 crackers	1	1 starch
RyKrisp®, all varieties	3 crackers	1	1 starch
Saltines	6 crackers	1	1 starch
Snack Sticks, all varieties	8 crackers	1	1 starch, 1 fat
Sociables®	8 crackers	1	1 starch, 1 fat
Toasted snack crackers, all varieties	8 crackers	1	1 starch, 1 fat
Town House®	8 crackers	1	1 starch, 1½ fat
Triscuit®	6 crackers	1	1 starch, 1 fat
Uneeda® biscuits	5 crackers	1	1 starch, 1 fat
Waverly® wafers	6 crackers	1	1 starch, 1 fat
Wheat Thins®	14 crackers	1	1 starch, 1 fat
Whole wheat crackers	4–6 crackers (1 oz)	1	1 starch, 1 fat
Whole wheat crackers, no fat added	2–5 crackers (¾ oz)	1	1 starch
Zweibach	3 crackers (¾ oz)	1	1 starch
Croissant			
Medium	1 croissant	1½	1½ starch, 2½ fat
Small	1 croissant	1	1 starch, 1½ fat
Croutons	1 cup	1	1 starch
Crumpet	1 crumpet	1	1 starch
English muffin, all varieties	1 muffin	2	2 starch
Falafel, 2" across	3 patties	1	1 starch, 1 med. fat meat, 2 fat
Farfel, dry	3 Tbsp	1	1 starch
Flour	3 Tbsp	1	1 starch
French toast	1 slice	1	1 starch, ½ med. fat meat
Grits, instant, plain or flavored	½ cup or 1 pkt	1	1 starch

Food	Quantity	Carbohydrate Choices	Exchanges
Hominy, cooked	½ cup	1	1 starch
Hummus	¼ cup	1	1 starch, 1 fat
Kasha (buckwheat groats)			
Cooked	½ cup	1	1 starch
Puffed	1 cup	1	1 starch
Lentils	½ cup	1	1 starch
Malanga, boiled	⅓ cup	1	1 starch
Marinara sauce	¾ cup	1	1 starch
Millet	¼ cup	1	1 starch
Miso	½ cup	2½	2½ starch, 1 med. fat meat
Muffin mix (as prepared)			
Apple streusel or wild blueberry	1/12 pkg	2	2 starch, 1 fat
Banana	1/12 pkg	1½	1½ starch, 1 fat
Wild blueberry or apple cinnamon, fat-free	1/12 pkg	2	2 starch
Muffins			
Apple cinnamon, banana nut, or blueberry	1 small (1½ oz)	1	1 starch, 1 fat
Carrot nut, chocolate chip, or oatmeal raisin	1 small (1½ oz)	1½	1½ starch, 1 fat
Oat bran or streusel	1 small (1½ oz)	1½	1½ starch, 1½ fat
Muffins, low-fat varieties	1 small (1½ oz)	1	1 starch
Noodles			
Cellophane	¾ cup	1	1 starch
Chinese	⅓ cup	1	1 starch
Chow mein	½ cup	1	1 starch, 1 fat
Ramen	½ pkg (1½ oz)	2	2 starch, 1½ fat
Ramen, low-fat	½ pkg (1½ oz)	3	3 starch
Somen, cooked	⅓ cup	1	1 starch
Spaetzle	⅓ cup	1	1 starch
Udon, cooked	⅓ cup	1	1 starch
Onion rings, frozen	4 rings	1	1 starch, 2 fat
Pancakes, frozen or microwave, 3½" across	2 cakes	1	1 starch, 1 fat
Pancakes (as prepared from mix)	3 cakes (4" across)	2	2 starch, 1 fat
Parsnips, cooked	½ cup	1	1 starch

Food	Quantity	Carbohydrate Choices	Exchanges
Pasta, cooked	½ cup	1	1 starch
Patty shell	1 shell	1	1 starch, 3 fat
Peas			
Green, cooked	½ cup	1	1 starch
Split, cooked	½ cup	1	1 starch
Plantain	½ cup	1	1 starch
Pocket/Pita bread			
4½" across	1 pocket/pita	1	1 starch
6½" across	½ pocket/pita	1	1 starch
Poi (taro), cooked	⅓ cup	1	1 starch
Polenta	⅓ cup	1	1 starch
Popcorn			
Air-popped	5 cups	1	1 starch
Microwave regular	3 cups	1	1 starch, 1 fat
Microwave low-fat or nonfat	3 cups	1	1 starch
Popover	1 small	1	1 starch, 1 fat
Potatoes			
Au gratin, homemade	½ cup	1	1 starch, 2 fat
Au gratin (as prepared from mix)	½ cup	1	1 starch, 1 fat
Baked or boiled	1 small (3 oz)	1	1 starch
Baked, with skin	1 medium (7 oz)	3	3 starch
Baked, without skin	1 medium (5½ oz)	2	2 starch
French-fried, frozen, oven-heated	10 strips	1	1 starch, 1 fat
French-fried, restaurant	10 strips	1	1 starch, 2 fat
Hash brown	½ cup	1	1 starch, 2 fat
Mashed	½ cup	1	1 starch
Potatoes O'Brien	½ cup	1	1 starch
Potato pancakes	1 cake	2	2 starch, 2 fat
Potato puffs, frozen, as prepared	½ cup	1	1 starch, 1 fat
Scalloped	½ cup	1	1 starch, 1 fat
Tater-Tots®	½ cup	1	1 starch, 1 fat
Twice-baked, frozen (5 oz)	½ potato	2	2 starch, 2 fat
Potato chips	12–18 chips (1 oz)	1	1 starch, 2 fat
Fat-free	12–18 chips (1 oz)	1	1½ starch

Food	Quantity	Carbohydrate Choices	Exchanges
Potato salad	½ cup	1	1 starch, 2 fat
Potato sticks or shoestrings	¾ cup	1	1 starch, 2 fat
Pretzels	¾ oz	1	1 starch
Mini	12 pretzels	1	1 starch
Very thin twisted	4 pretzels	1	1 starch
Very thin sticks	65 sticks	1	1 starch
Puppodums, plain	2 small	1	1 starch
Quinoa, cooked	⅓ cup	1	1 starch
Rice			
Basmati, cooked	½ cup	1	1 starch
Brown, cooked	⅓ cup	1	1 starch
Fried	⅓ cup	1	1 starch, 1 fat
Instant, cooked	⅓ cup	1	1 starch
Long-grain, cooked	⅓ cup	1	1 starch
White, cooked	⅓ cup	1	1 starch
Wild, cooked	½ cup	1	1 starch
Rice cakes, all flavors			
4" across	2 cakes	1	1 starch
Mini	½ oz	1	1 starch
Rice milk	½ cup	1	1 starch
Roll			
Brown and serve	1 small	1	1 starch
Crescent or twist	1 roll	1	1 starch, 1 fat
Dinner	1 small	1	1 starch
Hard	1 small	1	1 starch
Rutabaga	¾ cup	1	1 starch
Salsify or oyster plant	¾ cup	1	1 starch
Scrapple	2 slices (½" thick)	1	1 starch, 1 high fat meat
Snack Foods			
Bugles®, all varieties	30 chips (1 oz)	1	1 starch, 1½ fat
Cheetos®, regular varieties	1 oz	1	1 starch, 2 fat
Cheetos®, light	1 oz	1	1 starch, 1 fat
Chex Snack Mix®, all varieties	⅔ cup (1 oz)	1	1 starch, 1 fat
Fritos® corn chips, all varieties	~34 chips (1 oz)	1	1 starch, 2 fat

Food	Quantity	Carbohydrate Choices	Exchanges
Dinosaur Grahams®	1 large	1	1 starch
Doo Dads®	½ cup (1 oz)	1	1 starch, 1 fat
Granola bars, all varieties	1 bar	1½	1½ starch, 1 fat
Party Mix®	¼ cup	1	1 starch, 2 fat
Potato chips	12–18 chips	1	1 starch, 2 fat
Potato chips, fat-free	12–18 chips	1	1½ starch
Power Bar®	1 bar (2 oz)	3	3 starch
Sandwich crackers, cheese or peanut butter filling	3 crackers	1	1 starch, 1 fat
Sesame chips	¼ cup	1	1 starch, 2 fat
Teddy Grahams®	15 crackers	1	1 starch, ½ fat
Soups, canned or dehydrated (prepared with water unless otherwise noted)			
Bean with bacon	1 cup	1½	1½ starch, 1 fat
Bean with ham, chunky	1 cup	2	2 starch, 1 meat
Beef, chunky	1 cup	1	1 starch, 1 meat
Beef noodle	1 cup	1	1 starch
Black bean	1 cup	1	1 starch
Cheese	1 cup	1	1 starch, 2 fat
Chicken, chunky	1 cup	1	1 starch, 1 meat
Chicken noodle	1 cup	1	1 starch
Chicken rice	1 cup	1	1 starch
Chili beef	1 cup	1½	1½ starch, 1 fat
Clam chowder, Manhattan	1 cup	1	1 starch
Clam chowder, New England (prepared with milk)	1 cup	1	1 starch, 1 fat
Cream of asparagus	1 cup	1	1 starch, 1 fat
Cream of mushroom	1 cup	1	1 starch, 1 fat
Cream of potato	1 cup	1	1 starch, 1 fat
Lentil with ham	1 cup	1½	1½ starch, 1 fat
Minestrone	1 cup	1	1 starch
Minestrone, chunky	1 cup	1½	1½ starch

Food	Quantity	Carbohydrate Choices	Exchanges
Oyster stew (prepared with milk)	1 cup	1	1 starch, 1 fat
Pea, split, with ham	1 cup	2	2 starch, 1 lean meat
Pea, split, with ham, chunky	1 cup	1½	1½ starch, 1 lean meat
Ramen noodle, all regular varieties	½ pkg	2	2 starch, 1½ fat
Ramen noodle, low-fat	½ pkg	3	3 starch
Tomato	1 cup	1	1 starch
Tomato bisque	1 cup	1½	1½ starch
Tomato rice	1 cup	1½	1½ starch
Turkey, chunky	1 cup	1	1 starch, 1 meat
Turkey noodle	1 cup	1	1 starch
Vegetable, chunky	1 cup	1	1 starch, 1 fat
Vegetable, vegetarian	1 cup	1	1 starch
Vegetable with beef	1 cup	1	1 starch
Won ton soup	1 cup (2 won tons)	½	½ starch
Soybeans, cooked	½ cup	½	½ starch, 1 med. fat meat
Spaghetti sauce	½ cup	1	1 starch
	1 cup	1	1 starch, 1 fat
Squash, winter (acorn, butternut)	1 cup	1	1 starch
Stroganoff sauce (prepared with milk and water)	½ cup	1	1 starch, 1 fat
Stuffing mix, all varieties, as prepared	⅓ cup	1	1 starch, 1 fat
Succotash	½ cup	1	1 starch
Sweet potato			
Mashed	⅓ cup	1	1 starch
Raw	½ medium	1	1 starch
Taco shell, 6" across	2 shells	1	1 starch, 1 fat
Tapioca, dry	2 Tbsp	1	1 starch
Tempeh	½ cup	1	1 starch, 2 med. fat meat

Food	Quantity	Carbohydrate Choices	Exchanges
Tortilla chips	6–12 chips (1 oz)	1	1 starch, 2 fat
Light varieties	6–12 chips (1 oz)	1	1 starch, 1 fat
Baked varieties	9 chips (1 oz)	1½	1½ starch
Tortillas			
Corn, 6" across	1 tortilla	1	1 starch
Flour, 7–8" across	1 tortilla	1	1 starch
Flour, 10" across	1 tortilla	1½	1½ starch
Flour, 12" across	1 tortilla	2	2 starch
Tostada shell	2 shells	1	1 starch, 1 fat
Vegetables, mixed (peas and carrots)	1 cup	1	1 starch
Waffles, 4½" square	1 waffle	1	1 starch, 1 fat
Mini	4 waffles	1	1 starch, ½ fat
Reduced-fat, 4½" square	1 waffle	1	1 starch
Wheat bran	⅓ cup	1	1 starch
Wheat germ, toasted, plain	¼ cup	1	1 starch, 1 very lean meat
Yam, cooked	½ cup	1	1 starch

CHAPTER 11

Fruit and Vegetable Lists

There's something almost magical about fruits and vegetables and the promotion of health. While we don't know exactly what it is that makes them so helpful, we do know that eating five or more fruit and/or vegetable servings a day can lower your risk for many chronic diseases. Low in fat and high in fiber, vitamins, and minerals, fruits and vegetables are a delicious and important part of any meal plan.

Whether fresh, canned, dried, frozen, or as juice, fruits are excellent food choices. They are low in sodium, and they provide important amounts of vitamins A and C and potassium. Fresh fruits are always a good choice; they are satisfying and you can take them anywhere as healthy snacks. Servings of fresh fruits vary in size because of water content. Fruits with a high water content, such as strawberries and watermelon, have a larger portion size than fruits with a low water content, such as bananas and dried fruits.

When you shop for canned fruits, look for those that are packed in their own juice, in water, or in light syrup. These are better choices than fruits canned in heavy syrup, which contain added sugars. Choose 100 percent fruit juices to get the vitamins and minerals they contain. Avoid fruit "drinks," "ades," and "punches," which usually contain added sugars, little real juice, and fewer vitamins and minerals. Because of the fiber content, a serving of canned or fresh fruit is often more satisfying than a serving of fruit juice.

Along with fruits, meals would be very drab without the color, crispness, and flavor of vegetables. Vegetables grow in abundant variety, from A (asparagus) to Z (zucchini). They are generally low in calories but high in fiber, vitamins, and minerals. Most dark-green and deep-yellow vegetables excel as a source of vitamin A, and many dark-green vegetables also supply valuable amounts of vitamin C. Because of the many nutritional benefits vegetables offer, it is recommended that we eat at least two to three servings each day. Vegetables are listed in the carbohydrate group because they do contain carbohydrate, but in much smaller amounts than starches, fruits, or milk.

If you have diabetes, keep in mind that fruits will affect your blood glucose differently than vegetables. One serving of fruit contributes fifteen grams of carbohydrate and is one carbohydrate choice. One serving of vegetables contributes only five grams of carbohydrate and has little effect on your blood glucose.

One fruit serving has:

15 grams of carbohydrate

60 calories

One fruit serving is:

1 small to medium fresh fruit

½ cup canned fruit

¼ cup dried fruit

⅓–½ cup fruit juice

Weights given for fruits include skin, core, seeds, and rinds.

Vegetable List

Consider vegetables a free food, unless you eat more than three servings at one time. If you have the salad bar for lunch, or if you have a plate of cooked vegetables (about three servings) for dinner, count the vegetables as one vegetable or one carbohydrate choice. Normal serving sizes are considered free foods.

One vegetable serving has:

5 grams carbohydrate

2 grams protein

20–25 calories

One vegetable serving is:

½ cup cooked vegetables

½ cup vegetable juice

1 cup raw vegetables

FRUIT LIST

Food	Quantity	Carbohydrate Choices	Exchanges
Apple	1 small (4 oz) or ½ cup slices	1	1 fruit
Dehydrated, dried	4 rings (¼ cup)	1	1 fruit
Apple cider or juice	½ cup	1	1 fruit
Applesauce, unsweetened	½ cup	1	1 fruit
Apricot nectar	⅓ cup	1	1 fruit
Apricots	4 whole (5½ oz)	1	1 fruit
Canned	½ cup	1	1 fruit
Dried	8 halves	1	1 fruit
Asian pear, raw	1 medium	1	1 fruit
Banana	1 small (4 oz)	1	1 fruit
Blackberries	¾ cup	1	1 fruit
Canned in heavy syrup	½ cup	2	2 fruit
Blueberries	¾ cup	1	1 fruit
Canned in heavy syrup	½ cup	2	2 fruit
Wild	½ cup	1	1 fruit
Boysenberries, frozen, unsweetened	1 cup	1	1 fruit
Breadfruit, raw	⅛ medium	1	1 fruit
Cantaloupe	⅓ small melon (11 oz) or 1 cup cubes	1	1 fruit
Carambala; see Star fruit			
Carrot juice	¾ cup (6 oz)	1	1 fruit
Casaba melon	1½ cup cubed	1	1 fruit
Catawba juice	¾ cup	1	1 fruit
Cherimoya, raw	½ medium	1	1 fruit
Cherries			
Sour red, canned, light syrup pack	⅓ cup	1	1 fruit
Sweet, fresh	12 cherries (3 oz)	1	1 fruit
Sweet, canned, juice pack	½ cup	1	1 fruit
Crabapples	¾ cup	1	1 fruit

Food	Quantity	Carbohydrate Choices	Exchanges
Cranberry juice cocktail (Cranapple®, Cranraspberry®, etc.)	⅓ cup	1	1 fruit or 1 other carb
Reduced-calorie	1 cup	1	1 fruit or 1 other carb
Cranberry-orange relish	2 Tbsp	1	1 fruit
Currants, red and white, raw	1 cup	1	1 fruit
Dates	3 medium	1	1 fruit
Elderberries	½ cup	1	1 fruit
Feijoa	3 medium or ½ cup puree	1	1 fruit
Figs	1½ large or 2 medium (3½ oz)	1	1 fruit
Dried	1½ medium	1	1 fruit
Kadota, canned in heavy syrup	½ cup (5 pieces)	2	2 fruit
Fruit cocktail, canned, juice pack	½ cup	1	1 fruit
Fruit juice blends, 100% juice	⅓ cup	1	1 fruit
Fruit spreads			
Kraft® reduced-calorie	8 tsp	1	1 fruit or 1 other carb
Poiret® fruit spread	1 Tbsp	1	1 fruit or 1 other carb
Polaner® All Fruit®	4 tsp	1	1 fruit or 1 other carb
Smucker's®, light	8 tsp	1	1 fruit or 1 other carb
Smucker's®, low sugar	8 tsp	1	1 fruit or 1 other carb
Smucker's® Simply Fruit®	4 tsp	1	1 fruit or 1 other carb
Welch® Totally Fruit®	4 tsp	1	1 fruit or 1 other carb
Gooseberries	1 cup	1	1 fruit
Granadilla; see Passion fruit			
Grapefruit	½ fruit (11 oz)	1	1 fruit
Sections, canned	¾ cup	1	1 fruit
Grapefruit juice	½ cup	1	1 fruit
Grape juice	⅓ cup	1	1 fruit

Food	Quantity	Carbohydrate Choices	Exchanges
Grapes	17 small	1	1 fruit
Ground-cherries, raw	1 cup	1	1 fruit
Guava	1 medium	1	1 fruit
Canned in heavy syrup	8 pieces	1	1 fruit
Homli fruit	1 medium	1	1 fruit
Honeydew	1 slice or 1 cup cubes	1	1 fruit
Kiwifruit	1 medium	1	1 fruit
Kumquats, raw	5 medium	1	1 fruit
Lemon	3 medium	1	1 fruit
Lemon juice	1 cup	1	1 fruit
Lime	3 medium	1	1 fruit
Lime juice	1 cup	1	1 fruit
Loganberries	¾ cup	1	1 fruit
Loquats, raw	5–6 fruits	1	1 fruit
Lychees, litchis	½ cup or 10 medium	1	1 fruit
Mandarin oranges			
Canned in light syrup	½ cup	1	1 fruit
Canned in own juice	¾ cup	1	1 fruit
Mango, raw	½ fruit or ½ cup	1	1 fruit
Melon balls, frozen	1 cup	1	1 fruit
Mulberries	1 cup	1	1 fruit
Nectarines	1 small (5 oz)	1	1 fruit
Orange	1 small	1	1 fruit
Orange juice	½ cup (6½ oz)	1	1 fruit
Orange-grapefruit juice	½ cup	1	1 fruit
Papaya	½ or 1 cup cubes	1	1 fruit
Papaya nectar	⅓ cup	1	1 fruit
Passion fruit, raw	3 medium	1	1 fruit
Passion fruit juice	½ cup	1	1 fruit
Peach	1 medium (6 oz) or ¾ cup slices	1	1 fruit
Halves, canned, juice pack	2 halves or ½ cup	1	1 fruit
Slices, canned, juice pack	¾ cup	1	1 fruit
Peach nectar	½ cup	1	1 fruit
Pear	½ large (4 oz)	1	1 fruit
Canned, juice pack	2 halves or ½ cup	1	1 fruit

Food	Quantity	Carbohydrate Choices	Exchanges
Pear nectar	⅓ cup	1	1 fruit
Persimmons, raw	½ medium	1	1 fruit
Pineapple	¾ cup	1	1 fruit
Canned, juice pack	1½ slices or ½ cup	1	1 fruit
Pineapple juice	½ cup	1	1 fruit
Plums	2 small (5 oz)	1	1 fruit
Canned, juice pack	3 medium or ½ cup	1	1 fruit
Pomegranate, raw	½ medium	1	1 fruit
Prickly pear, raw	1½ medium	1	1 fruit
Pomelo, raw	¾ cup sections	1	1 fruit
Prune juice	⅓ cup	1	1 fruit
Prunes, dried	3 medium	1	1 fruit
Quince, raw	1 medium	1	1 fruit
Raisins	2 Tbsp	1	1 fruit
Raspberries	1 cup	1	1 fruit
Canned in heavy syrup	½ cup	2	2 fruit
Rhubarb, diced	2 cups	1	1 fruit
Sapodilla	1 medium	1	1 fruit
Sapota, raw	1 small	1	1 fruit
Star fruit (Carambola)	1½ medium	1	1 fruit
Strawberries	1¼ cup	1	1 fruit
Frozen, unsweetened	1 cup	1	1 fruit
Tamarinds, raw	12 small	1	1 fruit
Tangelos	1 medium	1	1 fruit
Tangerine juice	½ cup	1	1 fruit
Tangerines	2 small (8 oz)	1	1 fruit
Canned, juice pack	⅔ cup	1	1 fruit
Tomato juice	1½ cup	1	1 fruit
Ugli fruit	¾ cup	1	1 fruit
Watermelon	1 slice (13½ oz) or 1¼ cup cubes	1	1 fruit

VEGETABLE LIST

Food	Quantity	Exchanges
Artichoke		
Base and soft end of leaves, cooked	½ medium	1 veg
Heart, cooked	½ heart	1 veg
Jerusalem artichokes	¼ cup	1 veg
Asparagus	7 spears	1 veg
Bamboo shoots, cooked	½ cup	1 veg
Beets, cooked	½ cup	1 veg
Bell pepper	1 medium	1 veg
Bok choy (Chinese chard), canned	1 cup	1 veg
Borscht	½ cup	1 veg
Broccoli, cooked	1 medium stalk or ½ cup	1 veg
Brussels sprouts	3 sprouts	1 veg
Cabbage, boiled	½ cup	1 veg
Cactus leaves (Nopales)	1 medium leaf	1 veg
Carrot	1 large or 2 small	1 veg
Carrot juice	¼ cup	1 veg
Cauliflower	⅙ medium head	1 veg
Celery	2 medium stalks	1 veg
Chayote, cooked	½ medium or ½ cup	1 veg
Chinese cabbage, Nappa, raw	2 cups shredded	1 veg
Collards, boiled	½ cup	1 veg
Cucumber	⅓ medium	1 veg
Daikon, raw	1 cup	1 veg
Dandelion greens, cooked	½ cup	1 veg
Eggplant, cooked	1 cup cubes	1 veg
Green beans	½ cup	1 veg
Heart of palm	½ cup or 3 sticks	1 veg
Italian green beans	½ cup	1 veg
Jicama, raw	½ cup	1 veg
Kale, cooked	½ cup	1 veg
Kohlrabi, raw or cooked	½ cup	1 veg
Leeks, raw	½ cup	1 veg

Food	Quantity	Exchanges
Lettuce		
Iceberg	⅙ large head	1 veg
Leaf	3 cups shredded	1 veg
Mushrooms	8 medium	1 veg
Mustard greens, cooked	1 cup	1 veg
Okra, cooked	8 average pods or ½ cup	1 veg
Onions, cooked	½ cup	1 veg
Pea pods, cooked	½ cup	1 veg
Pumpkin, mashed	½ cup	1 veg
Radishes	5 medium	1 veg
Rhubarb	1 cup	1 veg
Rutabaga, cooked	½ cup	1 veg
Salsa dip	¼ cup	1 veg
Sauerkraut, canned	½ cup	1 veg
Snap beans, cooked	½ cup	1 veg
Snow peas, cooked	½ cup	1 veg
Spinach	1 cup raw or ½ cup cooked	1 veg
Creamed	½ cup	1 veg, 1 fat
Sprouts (alfalfa, bean, soybean)	1 cup raw or ¾ cup cooked	1 veg
Summer squash, cooked	½ cup	1 veg
Tomatillos	2 medium	1 veg
Tomato juice	½ cup	1 veg
Tomato	1 whole	1 veg
Paste	2 Tbsp	1 veg
Puree	¼ cup	1 veg
Sauce	⅓ cup	1 veg
Stewed	½ cup	1 veg
Turnip greens, cooked	½ cup	1 veg
Vegetable juice cocktail (V8®, Beefamato®, Clamato®, etc.)	½ cup	1 veg
Water chestnuts, canned	6 whole	1 veg
Wax beans	½ cup	1 veg
White mustard cabbage, cooked	½ cup	1 veg
Yard-long beans, cooked	4 pods	1 veg
Zucchini	1 medium	1 veg

CHAPTER 12

Milk List

The Milk List is relatively short but packed with good food choices. Milk and milk products give our bodies calcium, which helps build strong bones and teeth, and protein, which helps repair tissues. Milk and milk products such as yogurt also contain about twelve to fifteen grams of carbohydrate per serving. It's important to eat two to three servings from this list each day—two for most people and three for women who are pregnant or breastfeeding. Teenagers and young adults to age twenty-four need three servings as well.

One potential pitfall of foods on the Milk List is fat. A milk exchange includes only trace amounts of fat, but many foods on the list have additional fat exchanges because of their high fat content. Whole milk packs eight grams of fat in each eight ounce glass, along with 150 calories. Even 2% milk contains five grams of fat per serving and 120 calories. Skim milk contains no fat and only 90 calories and is the recommended choice for nearly everyone. However, 1% milk contains two and a half grams of fat per serving and is a good choice for people who dislike skim milk. Babies need the essential fatty acids found in whole milk, so they should not begin drinking skim or low-fat milk until they are two years old. If you are lactose intolerant or if you are following a vegan diet, soy milk and rice milk are good alternatives to cow's milk.

People often feel very attached to the type of milk they drink. People who drink whole milk usually don't like skim milk because they say it tastes like water, and skim milk fans don't like whole milk because to them it tastes like cream. But because the desire for fat is learned instead of innate, it is possible to get used to a lower-fat milk, no matter what type of milk you grew up drinking. If you currently drink whole milk, switch to 2% milk for a few months. After you've become used to it, try 1% milk and eventually skim milk.

Yogurt is an excellent milk choice. Nonfat or low-fat plain and artificially sweetened varieties are the best choices if you are trying to limit your sugar or calorie intake. An eight-ounce container of regular fruit-flavored yogurt can contain six to eight teaspoons of sugar (about forty-five grams of carbohydrate) and up to three grams of fat. Instead, try fruit-flavored yogurts sweetened with aspartame or another sugar substitute, or buy plain nonfat yogurt and flavor it yourself with fresh fruit or with unsweetened canned fruit or fruit juice.

As you scan the Milk List, you may wonder why cheese is not included. Though cheese is a milk product, it does not contain carbohydrate. Nutritionally, cheese is closer to meats; you can find it in the Meat and Meat Substitutes List in chapter 14.

One milk serving has:	One milk serving is:
12 grams carbohydrate	1 cup skim or 1% milk
8 grams protein	8 ounces plain, nonfat yogurt
trace amounts of fat	½ cup evaporated skim milk
90 calories	

MILK LIST

Food	Quantity	Carbohydrate Choices	Exchanges
Alba® cocoa mix, powder	~19 gm pkt	1	1 milk
Alba® Fit 'n Frosty®	~21 gm pkt	1	1 milk
Buttermilk, nonfat or low-fat	1 cup	1	1 milk
Chocolate milk, 1%	1 cup	1	1 milk
Cocoa/hot chocolate; *see* Other Carbohydrates List			
Evaporated milk			
Skim, canned	½ cup	1	1 milk
Whole, canned	½ cup	1	1 milk, 1 ½ fat
Filled milk	1 cup	1	1 milk, 1 fat
Goat's milk	1 cup	1	1 milk, 1 ½ fat
Instant breakfast; *see* Other Carbohydrates List			
Kefir	1 cup	1	1 milk, 1 ½ fat
Lactaid®	1 cup	1	1 milk

Food	Quantity	Carbohydrate Choices	Exchanges
Milk			
Skim milk	1 cup	1	1 milk
½% milk	1 cup	1	1 milk
1% milk	1 cup	1	1 milk, ½ fat
2% milk	1 cup	1	1 milk, 1 fat
Whole milk	1 cup	1	1 milk, 2 fat
Milk, nonfat dry	¼ cup dry mix	1	1 milk
Rice Dream®	1 cup	2	2 other carb
Soy milk	1 cup	1½	1½ milk, 1 fat
Light	1 cup	1	1 milk
Sweet acidophilus	1 cup	1	1 milk, 1 fat
Weight Watchers® shake mixes	1 envelope	1	1 milk
Yogurt			
Custard style, plain	1 cup (8 oz)	1½	1½ milk, 1 fat
Custard style, flavored	¾ cup (6 oz)	2	2 milk, 1 fat
Fruit-flavored	1 cup (8 oz)	3	1 milk, 2 other carb
Fruit-flavored, light	¾ cup (6 oz)	1	1 milk
Fruit-flavored, nonfat or low-fat with sugar substitute	1 cup (8 oz)	1	1 milk
Plain, low-fat	¾ cup (6 oz)	1	1 milk, 1 fat
Plain, nonfat	¾ cup (6 oz)	1	1 milk

CHAPTER 13

Other Carbohydrates List

Other carbohydrates are foods with appealing tastes but not much to offer nutritionally—foods like cakes, pies, cookies, jam, candy, and other sweets with added sugar. Typically high in fat and added sugars, these foods give us "empty calories" without other important vitamins and minerals. Nevertheless, people have a natural liking for sweet foods, so it's not surprising that most of us get cravings for chocolate and other sweets despite their dubious nutritional value. How do you handle these cravings and still stick to a healthy meal plan?

As in many things, moderation is the key. No one can eat large amounts of foods on this list and maintain weight, and people with diabetes cannot eat large amounts of these foods without elevating their blood glucose levels. However, vowing to give up sweets altogether may backfire—"all or nothing" diets seldom work over the long run and can lead to binges when they fail. It's wiser to allow yourself to indulge, but to set some boundaries on how much and how often. General guidelines for including foods from the Other Carbohydrates List are:

- When you do eat these foods, substitute them for starch, fruit, or milk exchanges (and fats, if necessary) in your meal plan rather than eating them in addition to your meal plan.

- Watch portion sizes carefully. In the lists you'll notice the portion sizes are often small.

- Try to limit your choices from this list to one per day.

If you've taken a trip down the cookie or cake aisle in recent years, you've probably noticed the low-fat, reduced-calorie versions of many desserts that have flooded supermarket shelves. Though these foods are fine if you watch portion sizes and exchanges closely, they are often misused. When a food is low-fat or light, people often ignore portion sizes and wind up eating much more than they should. And because low-fat or nonfat sweets don't taste as rich as the original versions, they may not even satisfy your craving. So if you really love chocolate chip cookies, you may be better off eating one really good cookie once or twice each week and skipping the low-fat substitutes.

If you have diabetes, you no longer need to consider foods on this list off limits. With carbohydrate counting, you can now substitute choices from this list for a starch, fruit, or milk choice on your meal plan. (Chapter 6 explains carbohydrate counting and how to make substitutions.) Some choices also will contain one or more fat servings. But as with everyone who is concerned with eating a balanced diet and staying healthy, you need to use caution and not make these substitutions too often.

One serving has:

15 grams carbohydrate

Varying amounts of protein, fat, and calories

One serving is:

1 unfrosted cake or brownie, 2" square

1 cookie, 3" across

2 small cookies

½ cup ice cream

½ cup frozen yogurt

OTHER CARBOHYDRATES LIST

Food	Quantity	Carbohydrate Choices	Exchanges
Bread pudding	½ cup	2½	2½ other carb, 1½ fat
Brownie, unfrosted	2" square	1	1 other carb, 1 fat
Cake			
Frosted	2" square	2	2 other carb, 1 fat
Unfrosted	2" square	1	1 other carb, 1 fat
Cake (as prepared from mix)			
Angel food cake, unfrosted	¹⁄₁₂ cake	2	2 other carb

Food	Quantity	Carbohydrate Choices	Exchanges
Applesauce spice cake, unfrosted	1/12 cake	2	2 other carb, 2 fat
Banana cake, unfrosted	1/12 cake	2	2 other carb, 2 fat
Carrot cake, unfrosted	1/12 cake	2	2 other carb, 1 fat
Gingerbread cake, unfrosted	1/12 cake	2	2 other carb, 1 fat
Candies, hard	3 average	1	1 other carb
Chocolate milk, low-fat	1 cup	2	2 other carb, 1 fat
Chocolate syrup	2 Tbsp	1	1 other carb
Chocolate wafers	3 wafers	1	1 other carb
Clearly Canadian® beverage	¾ cup (6 oz)	1	1 other carb
Cocoa/hot chocolate mix	3 Tbsp	1½	1½ other carb
No sugar added, reduced calorie	3 Tbsp	1	1 other carb
Fat-free	3 Tbsp	½	½ other carb
Cookies			
1¾" across	2 cookies	1	1 other carb, 1 fat
3" across	1 cookie	1	1 other carb, 1 fat
Animal crackers	8 cookies	1	1 other carb
Butter cookies	4 cookies	1	1 other carb, 1 fat
Chocolate chip cookies, 1¾" across	2 cookies	1	1 other carb, 1 fat
Dinosaur cookies, mini	14 cookies	1	1 other carb, ½ fat
Fig Newtons® or fig bars	2 cookies	1½	1½ other carb
Fortune cookies	2 cookies	1	1 other carb
Frookies®	2 cookies	1	1 other carb, 1 fat
Gingersnaps	3 cookies	1	1 other carb
Ladyfingers®	2 cookies	1	1 other carb
Lorna Doone® shortbread	6 cookies	1	1 other carb, 1 fat
Nilla® vanilla wafers	5 cookies	1	1 other carb, ½ fat

Food	Quantity	Carbohydrate Choices	Exchanges
Oatmeal or oatmeal raisin cookies	2 cookies	1	1 other carb, 1 fat
Oreo® sandwich cookies	2 cookies	1	1 other carb, 1 fat
Peanut butter cookies	2 cookies	1	1 other carb, 1 fat
Sandwich cookie with creme filling	2 small	1	1 other carb, 1 fat
Sugar cookies	2 small	1	1 other carb, 1 fat
Sugar wafers	2 cookies	1	1 other carb, 1 fat
Vanilla wafers	8 cookies	1½	1½ other carb, 1 fat
Cookies, fat-free	2 small	1	1 other carb
Corn syrup or honey	1 Tbsp	1	1 other carb
Cranberry sauce	¼ cup	2	2 other carb
Cream puff shell	1 small	1	1 other carb, 2 fat
Cupcake, frosted	1 small	2	2 other carb, 1 fat
Custard, baked	½ cup	1	1 other carb, 1 med. fat meat
Danish	1 medium (2½ oz)	2½	2½ other carb, 2 fat
Doughnut			
Glazed, 3¾" across	1 doughnut (2 oz)	2	2 other carb, 2 fat
Plain cake	1 medium (1½ oz)	1½	1½ other carb, 2 fat
Eggnog, nonalcoholic	½ cup	1	1 other carb, 2 fat
Frozen yogurt			
Low-fat or fat-free	⅓ cup	1	1 other carb
Fat-free, no sugar added	½ cup	1	1 other carb
Fruit and cream bar, frozen	1 bar	1	1 other carb
Fruit ice	¼ cup	1	1 other carb
Fruit juice bar, 100% juice	1 bar	1	1 other carb
Fruit Roll-Up®	1 (½ oz)	1	1 other carb
Fruit snacks, chewy	1 roll (¾ oz)	1	1 other carb

Food	Quantity	Carbohydrate Choices	Exchanges
Fruit spreads	1 Tbsp	1	1 other carb
Gatorade®	1 cup	1	1 other carb
Gelatin, regular	½ cup	1	1 other carb
Gelatin desserts	½ cup	1	1 other carb
Granola bars	1 bar	1	1 other carb, 1 fat
Fat-free	1 bar	2	2 other carb
Gumdrops	18 average	1	1 other carb
Hawaiian Punch®, reduced-calorie	1 cup	1	1 other carb
Honey	1 Tbsp	1	1 other carb
Ice cream, all flavors	½ cup	1	1 other carb, 2 fat
Light	½ cup	1	1 other carb, 1 fat
Fat-free, no sugar added	½ cup	1	1 other carb
Ice cream bar	1 bar	1	1 other carb, 2 fat
No sugar added	1 bar	1	1 other carb, 2 fat
Ice cream sandwich	1 sandwich	2	2 other carb, 1 fat
No sugar added	1 sandwich	1½	1½ other carb, 1 fat
Instant Breakfast®, fat-free			
Mix only	1 pkg dry	2	2 other carb
Prepared with skim milk	1 pkg + 1 cup milk	2	1 milk, 1 other carb
Instant Breakfast®, fat-free no sugar added			
Mix only	1 pkg dry	1	1 other carb
Prepared with skim milk	1 pkg + 1 cup milk	2	1 milk, 1 other carb
Jam or jelly, regular	1 Tbsp	1	1 other carb
Jelly beans	9 candies	1	1 other carb
Lemon drops	8 candies	1	1 other carb
Lemonade, punch, or fruit drink	½ cup	1	1 other carb
LifeSavers®	8 candies	1	1 other carb
Marshmallows	3 large	1	1 other carb
New York Seltzer®	¾ cup (6 oz)	1	1 other carb

Food	Quantity	Carbohydrate Choices	Exchanges
Pie			
Fruit with 2 crusts	⅙ pie	3	2 other carb, 1 fruit, 2 fat
Pumpkin or custard	⅛ pie	1	1 other carb, 2 fat
Pie crust	⅙ crust	1	1 other carb, 2 fat
Pound cake, unfrosted	½" slice	1½	1½ other carb, 1 fat
Pudding (all flavors)			
Regular (prepared with skim milk)	½ cup	2	2 other carb, 1 fat
Sugar-free (prepared with skim milk)	½ cup	1	1 other carb
Pudding pops, frozen	1 pop	1	1 other carb
Rice pudding	½ cup	2	2 other carb, 1 fat
Salad dressing, fat-free	¼ cup	1	1 other carb
Sherbet	¼ cup	1	1 other carb
Shortcake, 3" across	1 cake	1	1 other carb
Snapple® beverage	¾ cup (6 oz)	1	1 other carb
Snap-Up® beverage	¾ cup (6 oz)	1	1 other carb
Soft drinks (soda pop), regular	¾ cup (6 oz)	1	1 other carb
Sorbet	¼ cup	1	1 other carb
Sugar, granulated	4 tsp	1	1 other carb
Sundance® sparkling mineral water, juice added	5 oz	1	1 other carb
Sweet roll	1 (2½ oz)	2½	2½ other carb, 2 fat
Syrup, maple	1 Tbsp	1	1 other carb
	¼ cup	4	4 other carb
Light	2 Tbsp	1	1 other carb
Tapioca pudding	½ cup	2	2 other carb, 1 fat
Tropicana® sparkling mineral water, juice added	5 oz	1	1 other carb
Yogurt, low-fat fruited	1 cup	3	2 other carb, 1 milk

PART FOUR

Meat, Fat, and Other Exchange Lists

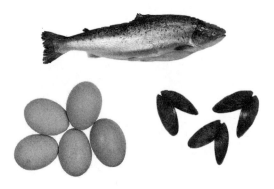

CHAPTER 14

Meat and Meat Substitutes List

Foods on the Meat and Meat Substitutes List are important sources of protein, which helps our bodies form new tissue, repair damaged tissue, and maintain healthy skin, muscles, and blood. Meat and meat substitutes include red meat, poultry, and fish, as well as other foods that are nutritionally similar to meats—cheese, eggs, nuts, and dried peas, beans, and lentils. Beans, peas, and lentils are on both the starch and meat lists because they contain both carbohydrate and a significant amount of protein. Most people need about two to three small servings of meat or meat substitute daily, or about six ounces (six exchanges).

All foods in the Meat and Meat Substitutes List contribute seven grams of protein per serving, but the amount of fat they contain varies. Meats and meat substitutes are divided into four lists based on the amount of fat they contain: very lean, lean, medium-fat, and high-fat. If a one-ounce portion of meat has more than ten grams of fat, it also will include fat exchanges. One of the great things about dried beans, peas, and lentils as a protein source is that you also get nutrients and fiber, and you don't get the fat.

Type of Meat Choice	Examples (see lists for portion sizes)
Very lean meat choice	White meat of turkey or chicken without skin; fresh or frozen fish; shellfish; nonfat processed meats and cheeses; cooked dried beans, peas, or lentils
Lean meat choice	Dark meat of poultry without skin; lean beef (round, sirloin, flank steak), processed ham, veal, cottage cheese; cheeses and processed meats with three grams or less fat per ounce

Medium-fat meat choice	Most beef and pork; poultry with skin, cheese and processed meats with four to five grams of fat per ounce; eggs
High-fat meat choice	Fried meats, poultry, or fish; prime cuts of beef, spareribs, processed meats; sausages; hot dogs; cheeses with approximately eight grams of fat per ounce; peanut butter

Here are some ways to include foods from this list in your meal plan while keeping your fat intake at healthy levels:

- Choose most of your servings from the extra lean and lean meat groups. Fish, chicken, and turkey are good choices, as long as they're not fried. For beef, look for cuts with words *round* or *loin* in them; for lamb, remember the *leg*; and for veal, all cuts except the breast.

- Use cooking methods that don't add fat. Broil, bake, or grill instead of frying. Always trim any visible fat from meat before cooking, and remove the skin from chicken and turkey before eating.

- Watch your portion sizes. Think of meat choices as an accompaniment to starch and vegetable choices, not as the main entrée. A three-ounce serving of meat is about the size of a deck of playing cards.

- Choose low-fat or skim milk cheeses. A one-ounce serving of cheese is about a one-inch cube or one prewrapped cheese slice.

- Go vegetarian at supper at least once a week by substituting cooked dried beans or lentils for the meat you would usually use in a dish. For example, try using beans instead of beef in chili or tacos, or make a hearty lentil soup for your main dish.

- Use nuts, which are naturally high in fat, carefully. Nuts in very small quantities are counted as fat exchanges. See the Fat List for portion sizes. The fat contained in nuts is primarily monounsaturated, which is less damaging to blood vessels than saturated fat.

In this list, serving sizes are based on cooked meat with the fat and bones removed. This is in contrast to restaurant menus, where meat portions are based on the weight of the uncooked meat. Because meat portions are difficult to estimate, it is helpful to weigh the cooked meat to determine how much you should eat. This is especially important when preparing meats you have not used before.

Keep in mind that there is a difference between a meat exchange and an average meat serving size. One exchange equals only one ounce of meat, fish, or poultry; one ounce of cheese; or one egg. Most actual serving sizes for meat, fish, poultry, or cheese are between two and four ounces (two and four exchanges). A two-ounce serving is one small chicken leg or thigh or one-half cup cottage cheese or tuna. A three to four ounce serving (three to four exchanges) is one medium pork chop, one small hamburger (one-quarter pound before cooking), one-half of a whole chicken breast, or one unbreaded fish fillet.

One very lean meat serving has:

7 grams protein

0–1 grams fat

35 calories

One very lean meat serving is:

½ cup cooked beans

1 ounce turkey breast

1 nonfat hot dog

1 ounce cheese or processed meat with 1 gram or less fat

One lean meat serving has:

7 grams protein

3 grams fat

55 calories

One lean meat serving is:

1 ounce canned or cured ham

2 slices (1 oz) low-fat luncheon meat

1 ounce tenderloin tips

1 ounce cheese or processed meat with 3 or less grams of fat

One medium fat meat serving has:

7 grams protein

5 grams fat

75 calories

One medium fat meat serving is:

1 ounce pot roast or ground beef

1 ounce string cheese

1 ounce pork chop

1 ounce cheese or processed meat with 4–6 grams of fat

One high fat meat serving has:

7 grams protein

8 grams fat

100 calories

One high fat meat serving is:

1 ounce prime rib

1 ounce regular cheese or processed meat

1–2 tablespoons peanut butter

MEAT LIST

Food	Quantity	Exchanges
Bacon (20 slices/lb)	3 slices	1 high fat meat
Beans, dried, cooked	½ cup	1 starch, 1 very lean meat
	1 cup	2 starch, 1 lean meat
Beef		
Barbecue ribs	1 oz	1 high fat meat
Beef breakfast strips	2 slices (1 oz)	1 high fat meat
Beef jerky	½ oz	1 very lean meat
Blade steak or pot roast	1 oz	1 med. fat meat
Brisket	1 oz	1 high fat meat
Brisket, lean	1 oz	1 med. fat meat
Chipped beef	1 oz	1 very lean meat
Chuck, arm pot roast	1 oz	1 lean meat
Chuck steak or roast, boned, well-trimmed	1 oz	1 med. fat meat
Club steak	1 oz	1 med. fat meat
Corned beef	1 oz	1 med. fat meat
Corned beef brisket	1 oz	1 high fat meat
Cubed steak	1 oz	1 lean meat
Eye of round, USDA Select or Choice grade, roast and steak	1 oz	1 lean meat
Family steak	1 oz	1 lean meat
Filet mignon	1 oz	1 lean meat
Flank steak, USDA Select or Choice grade	1 oz	1 lean meat
Ground beef	1 oz	1 med. fat meat
Ground beef, drained	½ cup	3 med. fat meat
Ground round or sirloin, very lean (90% lean)	1 oz	1 lean meat
Hamburger, more than 20% fat	1 oz	1 high fat meat
Kabob cubes	1 oz	1 lean meat
Loin strip steaks	1 oz	1 lean meat
Meatballs	1 oz	1 med. fat meat
Meatloaf	1 oz	1 med. fat meat
New York strip steak	1 oz	1 med. fat meat
Porterhouse steak, trimmed of fat	1 oz	1 med. fat meat

Food	Quantity	Exchanges
Porterhouse steak, USDA Select or Choice grade	1 oz	1 lean meat
Prime rib or steak, untrimmed	1 oz	1 high fat meat
Prime rib, trimmed of fat	1 oz	1 med. fat meat
Rib roast	1 oz	1 med. fat meat
Rib roast, USDA Select or Choice grade	1 oz	1 lean meat
Roast beef, thin sliced	1 oz	1 very lean meat
Round bottom roast, USDA Select or Choice grade	1 oz	1 lean meat
Round tip roast and steak	1 oz	1 lean meat
Round top or London Broil steaks	1 oz	1 lean meat
Rump roast, USDA Select or Choice grade	1 oz	1 lean meat
Scallopini	1 oz	1 lean meat
Shank	1 oz	1 lean meat
Short ribs	1 oz	1 med. fat meat
Shoulder roast	1 oz	1 med. fat meat
Sirloin tip roast	1 oz	1 med. fat meat
Sirloin top steak, USDA Select or Choice grade	1 oz	1 lean meat
Skirt steak	1 oz	1 lean meat
Stew meat	1 oz	1 lean meat
Sweetbreads	1 oz	1 lean meat
T-bone steak	1 oz	1 med. fat meat
T-bone, USDA Select or Choice grade	1 oz	1 lean meat
Tenderloin steak	1 oz	1 lean meat
Tenderloin tips	1 oz	1 lean meat
Tenderloin, USDA Select or Choice grade	1 oz	1 lean meat
Tongue	1 oz	1 med. fat meat
Beefalo	1 oz	1 very lean meat
Beerwurst	1 oz	1 high fat meat
Bratwurst	1 link	2 high fat meat, 1 fat
Braunschweiger	1 link	1 high fat meat
Buffalo	1 oz	1 very lean meat
Capon	1 oz	1 lean meat

Food	Quantity	Exchanges
Caviar, black and red	2 Tbsp	1 med. fat meat
Cheese		
Alpine Lace Free 'n Lean® fat-free cheese	1 oz	1 very lean meat
Alpine Lace Free 'n Lean® cheese products	1 oz	1 lean meat
American cheese or American cheese food	1 oz	1 high fat meat
Blue cheese	1 oz	1 high fat meat
Borden® Lite-Line® cheeses	1 oz	1 lean meat
Brick	1 oz	1 high fat meat
Brie	1 oz	1 high fat meat
Camembert	1 oz	1 high fat meat
Caraway	1 oz	1 high fat meat
Cheddar	1 oz	1 high fat meat
Cheese ball or log	1 oz	1 high fat meat
Cheese spread	2 Tb	1 high fat meat
Colby	1 oz	1 high fat meat
Cold pack cheese food	1 oz	1 high fat meat
Cottage cheese, nonfat or low-fat	¼ cup	1 very lean meat
Cottage cheese, 4.5% fat	¼ cup	1 lean meat
Crystal Farm® light and reduced-fat cheeses	1 oz	1 lean meat
Edam	1 oz	1 high fat meat
Feta	1 oz	1 med. fat meat
Fontina	1 oz	1 high fat meat
Gjetost	1 oz	1 high fat meat
Gouda	1 oz	1 high fat meat
Gruyere	1 oz	1 high fat meat
Havarti	1 oz	1 high fat meat
Healthy Choice® fat-free cheese	1 oz	1 very lean meat
Kaukauna® Lite cheese product	1 oz	1 lean meat
Kraft® fat-free cheese	1 oz	1 very lean meat
Kraft® flavored spreads	1 oz	1 med. fat meat
Kraft light and low-fat singles	1 oz	1 lean meat
Kraft® Light 'n Lively®	1 oz	1 lean meat
Laughing Cow® low-fat	1 oz	1 lean meat

Food	Quantity	Exchanges
Lifetime® low-fat	1 oz	1 lean meat
Light Philadelphia® cream cheese	1 oz	1 med. fat meat
Light 'n Lively® varieties	1 oz	1 med. fat meat
Limburger	1 oz	1 high fat meat
Monterey Jack	1 oz	1 high fat meat
Mozzarella, natural (part skim)	1 oz	1 med. fat meat
Mozzarella, whole milk	1 oz	1 high fat meat
Muenster	1 oz	1 high fat meat
Neufchatel	1 oz	1 high fat meat
Parmesan, grated	2 Tbsp	1 lean meat
Parmesan, hard	½ oz	1 med. fat meat
Pimento	1 oz	1 high fat meat
Port du Salut	1 oz	1 high fat meat
Provolone	1 oz	1 high fat meat
Ricotta, low-fat	2 Tbsp (1 oz)	1 lean meat
Ricotta, natural	¼ cup (2 oz)	1 med. fat meat
Ricotta, whole milk	1 oz	1 high fat meat
Romano	½ oz	1 med. fat meat
Sargento® light string cheese	1 oz	1 lean meat
Sargento® pot cheese	1½ oz	1 lean meat
String cheese	1 oz	1 med. fat meat
Swiss or swiss cheese food	1 oz	1 high fat meat
Tilsit	1 oz	1 high fat meat
Weight Watchers® low-fat cheese slices	1 oz	1 lean meat
Weight Watchers® cream cheese spread	1 oz	1 lean meat
Weight Watchers® natural cheddar	1 oz	1 med. fat meat
Cheese, fat-free	1 oz	1 very lean meat
Chicken		
Breaded and fried	3 oz	1 starch, 3 med. fat meat, 1–2 fat
Canned	1 oz	1 lean meat
Chicken spread	2 Tbsp (1 oz)	1 med. fat meat
Dark meat, no skin	1 oz	1 lean meat
Dark meat, with skin	1 oz	1 med. fat meat

Food	Quantity	Exchanges
Diced chicken	¼ cup	1 very lean meat
Fried with skin	1 oz	1 med. fat meat
Giblets or gizzard	1 oz	1 lean meat
Ground chicken	1 oz	1 med. fat meat
Livers, simmered	4 average	1 lean meat
Nuggets	3 oz	1 starch, 2 med. fat meat, 1 fat
Patties, breaded, fried	3 oz	1 starch, 2 med. fat meat, 1 fat
Southern fried chicken	3 oz	1 starch, 2 med. fat meat, 2 fat
White meat, no skin	1 oz	1 very lean meat
White meat, with skin	1 oz	1 lean meat
Chitterlings	1 oz	1 high fat meat
Clams	4 small	1 very lean meat
Cocktail wieners	3 weiners	1 high fat meat
Cold cuts		
Barbecue loaf, pork and beef	2 slices (1 oz)	1 med. fat meat
Boiled ham	2 slices	1 lean meat
Bologna	1 oz	1 high fat meat
Corned beef loaf, jellied	1 oz	1 lean meat
Deli thin, shaved meats	1 oz	1 very lean meat
Ham and cheese loaf	1 oz	1 med. fat meat
Headcheese	1 oz	1 med. fat meat
Old-fashioned loaf	1 oz	1 med. fat meat
Olive loaf	1 oz	1 high fat meat
Pastrami	1 oz	1 high fat meat
Pickle & pimiento loaf	1 oz	1 high fat meat
Salami	1 oz	1 high fat meat
Summer sausage (thuringer)	1 oz	1 high fat meat
Turkey cotto salami	1 oz	1 med. fat meat
Turkey pastrami (3 grams or less fat per ounce)	1 oz	1 lean meat
Turkey summer sausage (3 grams or less fat per ounce)	1 oz	1 med. fat meat
Cold cuts, low-fat	2 slices	1 lean meat
Cornish hen, no skin	1 oz	1 very lean meat
Crab		
Blue and king, steamed	1 oz	1 very lean meat
Canned meat	¼ cup	2 very lean meat

Food	Quantity	Exchanges
Crab cakes	1 medium	2 lean meat
Crab Dungeness	1 oz	1 very lean meat
Crayfish	16 crayfish	1 very lean meat
Duck, well-drained of fat, no skin	1 oz	1 lean meat
Eggs	1 egg	1 med. fat meat
Egg omelet	2 eggs	2 med. fat meat, 1 fat
Egg substitutes, plain	¼ cup	1 very lean meat
Egg whites	2 egg whites	1 very lean meat
Falafel, 2" across	3 patties (2 oz)	1 starch, 1 med. fat meat, 2 fat
Fish		
Anchovy, drained	7 anchovies	1 med. fat meat
Catfish, baked or broiled	1 oz	1 lean meat
Cod, baked or broiled	1 oz	1 very lean meat
Fish sticks	4 sticks	1 starch, 1 med. fat meat
Flounder, baked or broiled	1 oz	1 very lean meat
Fried fish	1 oz	1 med. fat meat
Haddock, baked or broiled	1 oz	1 very lean meat
Halibut, baked or broiled	1 oz	1 very lean meat
Herring, uncreamed or smoked	1 oz	1 lean meat
Mackerel (Atlantic, Pacific, Jack), baked or broiled	1 oz	1 med. fat meat
Ocean perch, baked or broiled	1 oz	1 very lean meat
Orange roughy, baked or broiled	1 oz	1 very lean meat
Pollock, baked or broiled	1 oz	1 very lean meat
Rainbow trout, baked or broiled	1 oz	1 very lean meat
Rockfish, baked or broiled	1 oz	1 very lean meat
Salmon (Atlantic or coho)	1 oz	1 lean meat
Salmon, pink, canned in water	1 oz	1 very lean meat
Salmon, red, canned	1 oz	1 lean meat
Sole, baked or broiled	1 oz	1 very lean meat
Tuna, canned in oil, drained	1 oz	1 lean meat
Tuna, canned in water	1 oz	1 very lean meat

Food	Quantity	Exchanges
Tuna, fresh, baked or broiled	1 oz	1 very lean meat
Walleye pike, baked or broiled	1 oz	1 very lean meat
Whiting, baked or broiled	1 oz	1 very lean meat
Franks		
Regular (beef or pork, 10/lb)	1 frank	1 high fat meat, 1 fat
Light (chicken, turkey, beef, or pork,10/lb)	1 frank	1 high fat meat
Fat-free (10/lb)	1 frank	1 very lean meat
Frog legs	3 medium	1 very lean meat
Goose, well-drained of fat, no skin	1 oz	1 lean meat
Ham salad or ham and cheese spread	2 Tbsp (1 oz)	1 med. fat meat
Ham		
Boneless smoked	1 oz	1 lean meat
Canned or cured	1 oz	1 lean meat
Country style	1 oz	1 high fat meat
Fresh	1 oz	1 lean meat
Minced	1 oz	1 med. fat meat
Hot dogs; *see* Franks		
Knockwurst	1 oz	1 high fat meat
Lamb		
Chops, sirloin or small loin	1 oz	1 lean meat
Cubes, stew	1 oz	1 lean meat
Ground	1 oz	1 med. fat meat
Leg of lamb, whole or boneless	1 oz	1 lean meat
Loin roast	1 oz	1 lean meat
Rib roast	1 oz	1 med. fat meat
Shish kebob	1 oz	1 lean meat
Shoulder roast	1 oz	1 lean meat
Sirloin roast	1 oz	1 lean meat
Lentils, dried, cooked	½ cup	1 starch, 1 very lean meat
Liver (high in cholesterol)	1 oz	1 lean meat
Liverwurst	1 oz	1 high fat meat
Lobster	1 oz	1 very lean meat
Miso	½ cup	2½ starch, 1 med. fat meat

Food	Quantity	Exchanges
Mussels	1 oz	1 very lean meat
Nuts		
Almonds	24 (1 oz)	1 med. fat meat, 2 fat
Cashews	18 (1 oz)	1 med. fat meat, 2 fat
Filberts (Hazelnuts)	12 (1 oz)	1 med. fat meat, 2 fat
Mixed nuts, dry or oil roasted	¼ cup (1 oz)	1 med. fat meat, 2 fat
Peanuts	¼ cup (1 oz)	1 med. fat meat, 2 fat
Pistachios	47 (1 oz)	1 med. fat meat, 2 fat
Nut butters		
Almond butter or almond paste	1 Tbsp	1 high fat meat or 2 fat
Peanut butter, creamy or chunky	1 Tbsp	1 high fat meat or 1 med. fat meat, 1 fat
	2 Tbsp	1 high fat meat, 1 fat or 1 med. fat meat, 2 fat
Sesame butter (tahini)	1 Tbsp	1 high fat meat
Octopus	1 oz	1 very lean meat
Ostrich	1 oz	1 very lean meat
Oysters, steamed	6 medium	1 lean meat
Oysters, breaded and fried	3 oz	1 starch, 1 med. fat meat, 1 fat
Pâte, chicken liver	1 oz	1 med. fat meat
Peas, dried, cooked	½ cup	1 starch, 1 very lean meat
Pheasant, no skin	1 oz	1 very lean meat
Pork; *see also* Bacon; Chitterlings; Ham		
Arm, picnic, roasted or cured	1 oz	1 med. fat meat
Barbecue ribs	1 oz	1 high fat meat
Boston butt	1 oz	1 med. fat meat
Breakfast strips	2 slices	1 high fat meat
Canadian-style bacon	1 oz	1 lean meat
Center loin chop	1 oz	1 lean meat
Chop	1 oz	1 med. fat meat
Country ribs	1 oz	1 high fat meat

Food	Quantity	Exchanges
Cutlet	1 oz	1 med. fat meat
Ground pork	1 oz	1 high fat meat
Headcheese	1 oz	1 med. fat meat
Loin blade	1 oz	1 med. fat meat
Loin roast, boneless	1 oz	1 lean meat
Rib chop	1 oz	1 lean meat
Rib roast, boneless	1 oz	1 lean meat
Rump, roasted	1 oz	1 med. fat meat
Shank, roasted	1 oz	1 med. fat meat
Shoulder, roasted	1 oz	1 med. fat meat
Sirloin chop, boneless	1 oz	1 lean meat
Sirloin roast	1 oz	1 lean meat
Spareribs	1 oz	1 high fat meat
Tenderloin	1 oz	1 lean meat
Top loin chop, boneless	1 oz	1 lean meat
Quail	1 oz	1 very lean meat
Pepperoni	1 oz	1 high fat meat
Pig's feet, cured, pickled	1 oz	1 high fat meat
Rabbit	1 oz	1 lean meat
Sausage		
Blood sausage (blood pudding)	1 oz	1 high fat meat
Chorizo	1 link	2 high fat meat, 1 fat
Kielbasa (with 3 or less fat per ounce)	1 oz	1 lean meat
Liver sausage	1 oz	1 high fat meat
Polish sausage	1 oz	1 high fat meat
Pork sausage, cooked	2 links or 1 patty	1 high fat meat
Smoked link sausage	1 link	1 high fat meat
Vienna sausage, regular	4 links (2 oz)	1 high fat meat, 1 fat
Vienna sausage (with 1 gram or less fat per ounce)	1 oz	1 very lean meat
Vienna sausage (with approximately 5 grams of fat per ounce)	1 oz	1 med. fat meat
Scallops, broiled	2 large or 5 small	1 very lean meat
Scrapple	1 slice (½" thick)	½ starch, ½ high fat meat
Seafood or shellfish, imitation	1 oz	1 very lean meat

Food	Quantity	Exchanges
Seeds		
Pumpkin or squash	¼ cup (1 oz)	1 med. fat meat, 2 fat
Sunflower	¼ cup (1 oz)	1 med. fat meat, 2 fat
Watermelon	95 (1 oz)	1 med. fat meat, 2 fat
Shrimp		
Boiled	1 oz	1 very lean meat
Breaded, fried	12 shrimp (4 oz)	1 starch, 3 med. fat meat
Soy milk	1 cup	1½ other carb, 1 med. fat meat
Soy protein, textured	1 cup	1 starch, 3 very lean meat
Soynuts	½ oz	1 lean meat
Spam®	1 oz	1 high fat meat
Squab (pigeon)	1 oz	1 lean meat
Squid	1 oz	1 very lean meat
Squirrel, roasted	1 oz	1 very lean meat
Tempeh	¼ cup	1 med. fat meat
Tofu	½ cup (2¼" block)	1 med. fat meat
Turkey		
Dark meat, no skin	1 oz	1 lean meat
Ground turkey	1 oz	1 med. fat meat
Smoked breast	1 oz	1 very lean meat
Turkey ham (with 1 gram or less fat per ounce)	1 oz	1 very lean meat
White meat, no skin	1 oz	1 very lean meat
Veal		
Chop, loin or sirloin	1 oz	1 lean meat
Cubes for kabobs	1 oz	1 lean meat
Cutlet	1 oz	1 lean meat
Cutlet, ground or cubed, unbreaded	1 oz	1 med. fat meat
Roast	1 oz	1 lean meat
Scallopine	1 oz	1 lean meat
Steak cutlet	1 oz	1 lean meat
Stew cubes	1 oz	1 lean meat
Venison	1 oz	1 very lean meat

Wieners; *see* Cocktail weiners; Franks

CHAPTER 15

Fat List

Researchers have long informed us that reducing the amount of fat in our diets can help prevent a host of health problems, from obesity to heart disease to cancer. It is recommended that we limit the amount of fat we eat each day to about thirty percent or less of our total calories. For a person eating 1800 calories a day, this is about sixty grams of fat; for a person eating 2500 calories a day, this is about eighty grams of fat. Half of this fat will occur naturally in some foods you eat, such as meat. The other half is from fats you add to your foods, and these are on the Fat List. Most meal plans include four to six fat exchanges each day. (Chapter 4 suggests some ways to cut back on the amount of fat in your diet.)

The Fat List is divided into three types of fat: saturated fat, monounsaturated fat, and polyunsaturated fat. Saturated fats such as lard, butter, coconut oil, palm oil, and palm kernel oil are associated with high blood cholesterol levels, and a diet high in saturated fat can raise your risk of heart disease and cancer. Monounsaturated fats such as olive oil or canola oil, on the other hand, have been linked with positive health benefits; they can lower the body's level of harmful LDL-cholesterol while preserving HDL-cholesterol, which helps protect against heart disease. This does not mean that you need to eat more monounsaturated fat than you do now. It does mean that it's wise to choose most of your fat servings from the monounsaturated and polyunsaturated sections of the list. A quick way to tell the difference between the different types of fat is that saturated fats are usually solid at room temperature, while the monounsaturated and polyunsaturated fats are usually liquid at room temperature.

You may notice that bacon, nuts, and peanut butter are included on this list as well as on the Meat and Meat Substitutes List. When used in small amounts, these foods are counted as fat choices. When used in larger amounts, they contain enough protein to be counted as high-fat meat choices. If you are using larger portions of these foods, count them as high-fat meat choices in your meal plan.

Fat-free salad dressings are counted as other carbohydrates or free foods, depending on the amount you eat. Fat-free products such as margarines, salad dressings, mayonnaise, sour cream, and cream cheese; nondairy coffee creamers and whipped toppings (used in small amounts) and nonstick cooking spray are also on the Free Foods List.

One serving has:

5 grams fat

45 calories

One serving is:

1 teaspoon margarine, butter, mayonnaise, or oil

1 tablespoon reduced-fat or light margarine or mayonnaise

1 tablespoon regular salad dressing

2 tablespoons reduced-fat or light salad dressing

2 tablespoons sour cream

3 tablespoons reduced-fat or light sour cream

FAT LIST

Food	Quantity	Exchanges
Monounsaturated Fats		
Almond butter	1 tsp	1 fat
Avocado	2 Tbsp mashed (⅛ or 1 oz)	1 fat
Nuts		
Almonds	6 nuts	1 fat
Brazil nuts	2 medium	1 fat
Cashews	6 nuts	1 fat
Chopped nuts	1 Tbsp	1 fat
Hazelnuts (Filberts)	5 nuts	1 fat
Macadamia nuts	3 nuts	1 fat
Peanuts	10 nuts (⅓ oz)	1 fat
Pecans	4 halves	1 fat

Food	Quantity	Exchanges
Pine nuts, pignolia	25 nuts (1 Tbsp)	1 fat
Pistachios	15 nuts	1 fat
Soynuts	1 oz	1 fat
Nuts, mixed	5–6 nuts	1 fat
Oil (canola, olive, peanut, macadamia, grapeseed, avocado, walnut)	1 tsp	1 fat
Olives		
Green, stuffed	10 large	1 fat
Ripe, black	8 large	1 fat
Peanut butter, smooth or crunchy	1 tsp	1 fat
Sesame seeds	1 Tbsp	1 fat
Tahini paste (sesame paste)	2 tsp	1 fat
Polyunsaturated Fats		
Margarine (stick, tub, or liquid)	1 tsp	1 fat
Reduced-fat or light	1 Tbsp	1 fat
Fat-free	1 Tbsp	free
Whipped	2 tsp	1 fat
Mayonnaise	1 tsp	1 fat
Reduced-fat or light	1 Tbsp	1 fat
Miracle Whip® salad dressing	2 tsp	1 fat
Reduced-fat or light	1 Tbsp	1 fat
Oil (corn, safflower, or soybean)	1 tsp	1 fat
Salad dressings	1 Tbsp	1 fat
Reduced-fat or light	2 Tbsp	1 fat
Blue-cheese, regular	2 tsp	1 fat
Blue-cheese, reduced-fat or light	1 Tbsp	1 fat
French	1 Tbsp	1 fat
Italian	1 Tbsp	1 fat
Ranch	1 Tbsp	1 fat
Thousand Island or Russian	2 tsp	1 fat
Vinegar and oil	2 tsp	1 fat
Seeds		
Pumpkin or squash	1 Tbsp	1 fat
Soybean	1 Tbsp	1 fat
Sunflower seed kernels	1 Tbsp	1 fat
Tartar sauce	2 tsp	1 fat
Walnuts	4 halves (1 Tbsp)	1 fat

Food	Quantity	Exchanges
Saturated Fats		
Anchiote, prepared	1 tsp	1 fat
Bacon, cooked (20 slices/lb)	1 slice	1 fat
Bacon grease	1 tsp	1 fat
Butter, stick or tub	1 tsp	1 fat
Reduced-fat stick or tub	1 Tbsp	1 fat
Whipped	2 tsp	1 fat
Cheese sauce	2 Tbsp	1 fat
Cheese spread	1 Tbsp	1 fat
Chicken fat	1 tsp	1 fat
Chitterlings, boiled	2 Tbsp (½ oz)	1 fat
Coconut, shredded	2 Tbsp	1 fat
Coffee whiteners		
Nondairy liquid	2 Tbsp	1 fat
Nondairy powdered	4 tsp	1 fat
Cream, half and half	2 Tbsp	1 fat
Cream cheese	1 Tbsp (½ oz)	1 fat
Reduced-fat or light	2 Tbsp (1 oz)	1 fat
Dips		
Cream cheese-based	1 Tbsp	1 fat
Light	¼ cup	1 fat
Sour cream-based	2 Tbsp	1 fat
Gravy		
Canned	¼ cup	1 fat
Mix (as prepared)	½ cup	1 fat
Lard	1 tsp	1 fat
Liver pâte, chicken	2 Tbsp	1 fat
Neufchatel	1 ½ Tbsp (¾ oz)	1 fat
Shortening	1 tsp	1 fat
Sour cream	2 Tbsp	1 fat
Reduced-fat or light	3 Tbsp	1 fat
Whipped toppings		
Frozen	3 Tbsp	1 fat
Mix (as prepared)	5 Tbsp	1 fat

CHAPTER 16

Free Foods List

This list contains foods you can eat in addition to your meal plan without worrying about substituting or exchanging. Free foods are foods that aren't nutritionally significant—they have less than twenty calories per serving or less than five grams of carbohydrate in a serving.

The term "free foods" doesn't necessarily mean that you can eat unlimited amounts of the foods on the list. Calories are still important, which is why some of these foods have serving sizes. Foods listed with a serving size should be limited to a total of fifty to sixty calories per day, or a total of three servings per day. You can eat free foods listed without a serving size as often as you like.

One serving has:

20 calories or less per serving

5 grams or less carbohydrate per serving

FREE FOODS LIST

Food	Quantity	Exchanges
Bacon bits	1 tsp	free
Barbecue sauce	1 Tbsp	free
Bean dip	2 Tbsp	free
Bran, unprocessed	2 Tbsp	free
Brewer's yeast	2 tsp	free
Butter Buds®, dry	3 tsp	free
Candies		
Gummy bears, sugar-free	2 pieces	free
Hard candy, sugar-free	1 piece	free
Carbonated water, noncaloric	–	free

Food	Quantity	Exchanges
Carbonated water, low-calorie with fruit juice added	12 oz	free
Catsup	1 Tbsp	free
Chewing gum, sugar-free	2 pieces	free
bubble gum, sugar-free	1 piece	free
Chili sauce	1 Tbsp	free
Chocolate milk mix, sugar-free	1 heaping tsp	free
Club soda (not tonic or quinine water)	–	free
Cocktail sauce	1 Tbsp	free
Cocoa, dry powder, unsweetened	1 Tbsp	free
Cocoa mix, hot, no sugar added	1 Tbsp	free
Coffee	–	free
Coffee whiteners		
Nondairy liquid	1 Tbsp	free
Nondairy powdered	2 tsp	free
Light nondairy creamer	1 Tbsp	free
Coffee-Mate®, liquid	1 Tbsp	free
Cooking spray, nonstick	–	free
Cranberries, cooked without sugar	½ cup	free
Cream cheese, fat-free	1 Tbsp	free
Crystal Light® Bars (frozen)	1 bar	free
Dips, low-fat (French onion, ranch)	2 Tbsp	free
Gelatin, sugar-free, low-calorie	–	free
Gelatin, unflavored	–	free
Gravy		
Au jus	¼ cup	free
Canned	2 Tbsp	free
All others	2 Tbsp	free
Horseradish	3 Tbsp	free
Ice cream cones (Comet® cups or waffle cones)	1 cone	free
Iced tea, sugar-free	–	free
Iced tea, sugar-free (as prepared from mix)	–	free
Jams and Jellies		
Dietetic	under 20 calories	free
Low-sugar spreads	2 tsp	free
Light	2 tsp	free

Food	Quantity	Exchanges
Spreadable fruit (All-Fruit®, Simply Fruit®, Totally Fruit®, etc.)	1 tsp	free
Kool-Aid® or other powdered drink mix, sugar-free	–	free
Lemon juice	–	free
Lime juice	–	free
Margarine		
Reduced-fat	1 tsp	free
Fat-free	1 Tbsp	free
Mayonnaise		
Reduced-fat	1 tsp	free
Fat-free	1 Tbsp	free
Mineral water, noncaloric	–	free
Miracle Whip®		
Reduced-fat	1 tsp	free
Fat-free	1 Tbsp	free
Molly McButter® sprinkles	2 tsp	free
Mrs. Dash® herb and spice blends	1 tsp	free
Mustard	1 Tbsp	free
Onions	–	free
Picante sauce	2 Tbsp	free
Pickle relish	1 Tbsp	free
Pickles, dill (not sweet)		
Large	1 ½ large	free
Small	–	free
Pimiento	–	free
Popsicles®, sugar-free	1 pop	free
Postum® beverage	2 tsp	free
Salad dressings		
Fat-free	1 Tbsp	free
Fat-free Italian	2 Tbsp	free
Salsa, all varieties	¼ cup	free
Sauerkraut	½ cup	free
Soft drinks (soda pop), diet	–	free
Soups		
Beef broth	1 cup	free
Chicken broth	½ cup	free
Consommé	¾ cup	free

Food	Quantity	Exchanges
Sour cream		
Fat-free	1 Tbsp	free
Reduced-fat or light	1 Tbsp	free
Soy sauce	1 Tbsp	free
Spices (garlic, basil, oregano, rosemary, thyme, etc.)	–	free
Steak sauce (Heinz 57®, A1®, etc.)	1 Tbsp	free
Sugar substitutes		
Equal® (aspartame)	–	free
Splenda((sucralose)	–	free
Sprinkle Sweet® (saccharin)	–	free
Sweet 'n Low® (saccharin)	–	free
Sweet One® (acesulfame K)	–	free
Sweet-10® (saccharin)	–	free
Sugar Twin® (saccharin)	–	free
Syrup		
Cary's® reduced-calorie	2 Tbsp	free
Sugar-free	2 Tbsp	free
Tabasco sauce	1 Tbsp	free
Taco sauce	1 Tbsp	free
Tang® beverage crystals, sugar-free	–	free
Tea, sugar-free	–	free
Teriyaki sauce	1 Tbsp	free
Tomato sauce	2 Tbsp	free
Vinegar	–	free
Wine used in cooking	–	free
Whipped topping		
Cool Whip®	2 Tbsp	free
Cool Whip® Light	2 Tbsp	free
Tonic water, sugar-free	–	free
Worcestershire sauce	1 Tbsp	free
Yogurt, nonfat	2 Tbsp	free

CHAPTER 17

Combination Foods List

Many foods are combinations of foods from several of the exchange lists—pizza, lasagna, and casseroles are a few popular examples. Combination foods have the advantage of giving you nutrients from many food groups at once, but it is sometimes hard to know how to use them in your meal plan. It's often difficult to know exactly which foods are in a mixed dish or casserole, and in what amounts.

The Starch List and Meat List can be used to count many combination foods. A good rule of thumb is to count one cup as two starch plus two medium fat meat. For example, one cup of either spaghetti and meat sauce, chili with beans, or macaroni and beef casserole is two starch and two medium fat meats. Depending on the ingredients, the casserole also may include a fat or a vegetable. One cup of tuna noodle casserole made with cream soup is two starch, two medium fat meat, and one fat.

The exchange values given below are averages; the exact exchanges in a dish vary depending on the amount of each ingredient in a particular recipe. Chapter 7 explains how to determine exchange values for your favorite recipes.

One serving is:	Exchanges for each item:
1 cup casserole	2 starch, 2 medium fat meat, 0–1 fat
1½ cup chili	2 starch, 2 medium fat meat
2 cups oriental entrée	2 starch, 1–2 vegetable, 1–2 medium fat meat
½ cup pasta salad or potato salad	1 starch, 1–2 fat
1 slice pizza, ⅛ large	1 starch, 1 vegetable, 1 medium fat meat, 0–1 fat
1 can (10¾ oz) chunky soup	1 starch, 1 vegetable, 2 medium fat meat

COMBINATION FOODS LIST

Food	Quantity	Carbohydrate Choices	Exchanges
Burrito, all varieties	1 (6 oz)	2	2 starch, 2 med. fat meat, 1 fat
Chicken à la king	1 cup	1	1 starch, 2 med. fat meat, 2 fat
Chicken and dumplings	1 cup	2	2 starch, 2 med. fat meat, 1 fat
Chicken and noodles	1 cup	2	2 starch, 2 med. fat meat, 1 fat
Chicken salad	½ cup	0	2 med. fat meat, 2 fat
Chili with beans	1 cup	2	2 starch, 2 lean meat
Chimichangas, all varieties	1 (6 oz)	2	2 starch, 1 med. fat meat, 3 fat
Chop suey	1 cup	1	1 starch, 3 med. fat meat
Chow mein (without noodles or rice)	2 cups	2	2 starch, 1 veg, 2 lean meat
Creamed chipped beef	1 cup	1	1 starch, 2 med. fat meat, 3 fat
Egg salad	½ cup	0	1 med. fat meat, 4 fat
Enchiladas	1 enchilada	2	2 starch, 1 med. fat meat, 1 fat
Fish cake, fried	3 pieces	1	1 starch, 3 med. fat meat
French toast	2 slices	2	2 starch, 1 med. fat meat, 1 fat
Entrée with less than 300 calories	1 (8 oz)	2	2 starch, 3 lean meat
Salisbury steak with gravy, roast beef or pork, mashed potatoes	1 (11 oz)	2	2 starch, 3 med. fat meat, 2 to 4 fat
Turkey or chicken with gravy, mashed potatoes, dressing	1 (11 oz)	2	2 starch, 2 med. fat meat, 2 fat
Hamburger Helper® main dishes	⅕ pkg, prepared	2	2 starch, 2 med. fat meat, 1 fat
Lasagna	1 cup	2	2 starch, 2 med. fat meat

Food	Quantity	Carbohydrate Choices	Exchanges
Macaroni and cheese	1 cup	2	2 starch, 1 high fat meat
Pasta salad	½ cup	1½	1½ starch, 1 to 2 fat
Pizza			
Cheese or sausage	1 small slice	1	1 starch, 1 med. fat meat
Cheese, thin crust	¼ of 10" (5 oz)	2	2 starch, 2 med. fat meat, 1 fat
Meat, thin crust	¼ of 10" (5 oz)	2	2 starch, 2 med. fat meat, 2 fat
Thick crust	¼ of 10"	4	4 starch, 1 med. fat meat, 1 fat
Pot pies, all varieties	1 average (7 oz)	3	3 starch, 1 med. fat meat, 4 fat
Potato salad	½ cup	1	1 starch, 1 to 2 fat
Quiche, all varieties	1 slice	1½	1½ starch, 2 med. fat meat, 2 fat
Ravioli			
Beef	1 cup	2½	2½ starch, 1 med. fat meat
Cheese	1 cup	2½	2½ starch, 1 high fat meat, 1 fat
Rice-A-Roni®	1 cup	4	4 starch, 2 fat
Salad; *see also* Chicken salad; Egg salad; Pasta salad; Potato salad			
Caesar salad	1 serving	0	2 veg, 6 fat
Chef salad (mixed greens, 3 Tbsp regular dressing, 1 oz cheese, chicken, or ham)	1 serving	1	3 veg (1 carbohydrate choice), 3 med. fat meat, 2 fat
Coleslaw	½ cup	0	1 veg, 2 fat
Waldorf salad	½ cup	0	1 fruit, 3 fat
Sandwiches			
Bacon, lettuce, tomato, mayonnaise	1 sandwich	2	2 starch, 3 fat
Chicken, lettuce, mayonnaise	1 sandwich	2	2 starch, 2 med. fat meat, 1 fat
Chicken salad sandwich	1 sandwich	2	2 starch, 2 med. fat meat, 1 fat

Food	Quantity	Carbohydrate Choices	Exchanges
Club sandwich (turkey or ham, bacon, tomato, lettuce and mayonnaise on 3 slices of bread)	1 sandwich	3	3 starch, 4 med. fat meat, 1 fat
Corned beef	1 sandwich	2	2 starch, 3 med. fat meat
Egg salad	1 sandwich	2	2 starch, 1 med. fat meat, 2 fat
Grilled cheese	1 sandwich	2	2 starch, 2 med. fat meat, 2 fat
Ham salad	1 sandwich	2	2 starch, 1 med. fat meat, 2 fat
Hot dog in roll	1 sandwich	1½	1½ starch, 1 high fat meat, 2 fat
Liverwurst	1 sandwich	2	2 starch, 1 high fat meat, 2 fat
Meat loaf	1 sandwich	2	2 starch, 3 med. fat meat
Peanut butter	1 sandwich	2	2 starch, 1 high fat meat, 1 fat
Roast beef or pork with gravy	1 sandwich	2	2 starch, 2 med. fat meat, 2 fat
Submarine sandwich or hoagie	1 large	4	4 starch, 4 med. fat meat, 1 fat
Tuna salad	1 sandwich	2	2 starch, 1 med. fat meat, 2 fat
Soufflé, cheese or spinach	1½ cup	½	½ starch, 2 med. fat meat, 1 fat
Soup			
Bean soup	1 cup	1	1 starch, 1 lean meat
Chicken noodle, vegetable beef, or other broth-type soup	1 cup	1	1 starch
Chunky soup	1 can (10¾ oz)	1	1 starch, 1 veg, 1 med. fat meat
Cream soups (prepared with water)	1 cup	1	1 starch, 1 fat
Split pea (prepared with water)	½ cup	1	1 starch
Tomato (prepared with water)	1 cup	1	1 starch

Food	Quantity	Carbohydrate Choices	Exchanges
Spaghetti with meatballs	1 cup	2	2 starch, 1 veg, 2 med. fat meat
Spanish rice	1 cup	3	3 starch, 1 fat
Stew, beef and vegetable	1 cup	1	1 starch, 2 med. fat meat
Tuna Helper® main dishes	⅕ pkg, prepared	2	2 starch, 2 med. fat meat
Tuna noodle casserole	1 cup	2	2 starch, 2 med. fat meat
Tuna salad	½ cup	0	2 med. fat meat, 1 fat

PART FIVE

Ethnic Exchanges

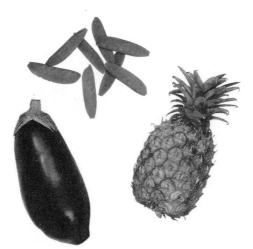

CHAPTER 18

Vegetarian Exchanges

Vegetarianism or near-vegetarianism has been practiced for thousands of years. People choose a vegetarian diet for many reasons—health, religious, philosophical, ecological, ethical, or economic. Others, while not giving up meat entirely, may decide to minimize their meat intake or to vary their diet with vegetarian meals from time to time. Whatever your motivation, if you have chosen or are considering a vegetarian way of eating, you'll find this chapter helpful.

There are several types of vegetarians. *Vegans*, or strict vegetarians, eat only foods from plant sources, such as fruits, grains, legumes (dried beans, peas, lentils), nuts, and seeds, and exclude all foods of animal origin. *Lactovegetarians* eat plant foods and dairy products but exclude meat, poultry, fish, and eggs. *Lacto-ovovegetarians* eat plant foods, dairy products, and eggs but exclude meat, poultry, and fish.

Traditional American meal planning is based on main dishes using meat, poultry, or fish. Vegetarians use alternative sources of protein from plants. In a vegetarian diet, legumes, grains, and soy products, such as tofu, supply most of the protein. Lacto-ovovegetarians may also get protein from eggs and dairy products.

All vegetarians, even vegans, can have healthy diets if they select a variety of foods and if they get enough calories to meet energy needs. In fact, vegetarian diets can offer many health benefits. Vegetarians tend to use more whole-grain products and legumes than nonvegetarians. Whole grains and legumes are excellent sources of fiber, vitamins, minerals, and protein. Meals with vegetable proteins in place of meat can be low in fat and cholesterol, provided high-fat dairy products such as cheese and whole milk are not eaten. A one-cup serving of cooked legumes has as much protein as a three-ounce portion of meat, fish, or poultry and contains little fat.

Protein is made up of about twenty amino acids. Of these amino acids, nine cannot be manufactured by the body. They are called *essential amino acids* because they must be supplied in the diet. Animal proteins such as meat and milk are called *complete proteins* because they supply all of the essential amino acids. Many plant proteins are lacking in one or more of the essential amino acids. However, foods that complement each other to create complete proteins are often naturally combined in a vegetarian diet. These complementary proteins do not necessarily need to be eaten at the same time; our bodies store essential amino acids from foods, which can be used to complement plant proteins eaten later.

In vegetarian meals, these foods are often eaten together and as a result become complete proteins:

- Lentils combined with grains (lentil soup with wheat bread)
- Legumes combined with grains (baked beans with brown bread)
- Legumes combined with rice (red beans and rice)
- Nuts combined with wheat (peanut butter on bread)

Plant proteins may also be combined with milk, yogurt, cheese, or egg to provide complete proteins. Some examples of these combinations are breakfast cereal and milk, or macaroni and cheese.

Unlike other plant proteins, soybeans and soy products are complete proteins by themselves and are comparable to meat. Soy products called meat analogs duplicate the taste and texture of foods such as steaks, chops, wieners, and hamburger. These products are convenient because they can be substituted for meat in meals without changing the rest of the menu. However, they are not essential for a well-balanced vegetarian diet.

Sample Lactovegetarian Menu

Menu	Exchanges
Breakfast	
Whole wheat toast, 2 slices	2 starch
Cooked oats, ½ cup	1 starch
Orange juice, ½ cup	1 fruit
Skim milk, 1 cup	1 milk
Margarine, 2 tsp	2 fat
Snack	
Apple, 1 medium	1 fruit
Lunch	
Hummus, ¼ cup	1 starch, 1 fat
Pocket bread, 1	1 starch
Yogurt, fruit-flavored, with sugar substitute, 1 cup	1 milk
Cottage cheese, ½ cup	2 lean meat
Diced tomatoes, shredded lettuce, diced onions, ½ cup	0–1 veg
Tahini, 2 tsp	1 fat
Snack	
Nonfat plain yogurt, 1 cup	1 milk
Fresh fruit, ½ cup	1 fruit
Dinner	
Spaghetti with lentil sauce, ½ cup pasta with 1 cup sauce	3 starch, 1 veg, 2 lean meat
Pineapple with juice, 1 slice	1 fruit
Green salad with sprouts, 1 small	1 veg
French dressing, 2 Tbsp	2 fat
Snack	
Popcorn, 3 cups	1 starch
Low-fat cheese, 1 oz	1 med. fat meat
Daily Total	
Exchanges:	9 starch, 4 fruit, 3 milk, 2–3 vegetable, 4 lean meat, 1 med. fat meat, 5 fat
Calories:	1800–1900
Carbohydrate:	245 grams (54%)
Protein:	90 grams (20%)
Fat:	50 grams (26%)

Sample Vegan Menu

Menu	Exchanges
Breakfast	
Rye toast, 2 slices	2 starch
Scrambled tofu, ½ cup	1 med. fat meat
Fresh fruit salad, 1 cup	2 fruit
Margarine, 2 tsp	2 fat
Snack	
Apple, 1 medium	1 fruit
Lunch	
Vegetable soup, 1 bowl	2 starch
Wheat roll, 1 small	1 starch
Tossed salad, 1 small	0–1 veg
Low-fat dressing, 2 Tbsp	1 fat
Snack	
Rice cakes, 4 cakes	2 starch
Almond butter, 1 tsp	1 fat
Dinner	
Pasta, 2 cups	4 starch
Primavera with broccoli, carrots, pea pods, ½–1 cup	1–2 veg
Steamed peas, ½ cup	1 starch
French bread, 1 slice	1 starch
Margarine, 1 tsp	1 fat
Snack	
Shake of soymilk and fruit, 1½ cups	1 milk, 1 fruit, 1 fat
Daily Total	
Exchanges:	13 starch, 4 fruit, 1 milk, 2–3 veg, 1 meat, 6 fat
Calories:	1800–1900
Carbohydrate:	285 grams (63%)
Protein:	60 grams (13%)
Fat:	50 grams (24%)

VEGETARIAN FOOD LIST

Food	Quantity	Carbohydrate Choices	Exchanges
Starch			
Amaranth, cooked	½ cup	1	1 starch
Arabic bread, Syrian bread loaf	½ of a 2-oz loaf	1	1 starch
Barley, cooked	⅓ cup	1	1 starch
Brewer's yeast	3 Tbsp	1	1 starch, 1 lean meat
Buckwheat flour, dark or light	3 Tbsp	1	1 starch
Buckwheat groats (kasha), cooked	½ cup	1	1 starch
Bulgur, cooked	½ cup (2 Tbsp dry)	1	1 starch
Carob flour	2 Tbsp	1	1 starch
Couscous, cooked	⅓ cup	1	1 starch
Falafel, 2" across	3 patties	1	1 starch, 1 med. fat meat, 2 fat
Hummus	¼ cup	1	1 starch, 1 fat
Millet, cooked	¼ cup	1	1 starch
Miso	3 Tbsp	1	1 starch
	½ cup	2½	2½ starch, 1 med. fat meat
Pasta	½ cup	1	1 starch
Pasta and tomato sauce	2 cups	4	4 starch, 2 veg, 1 fat
Pocket/Pita bread			
4½" across	1 pocket/pita	1	1 starch
6½" across	½ pocket/pita (1 oz)	1	1 starch
Rice			
Brown, cooked	⅓ cup	1	1 starch
White, cooked	⅓ cup	1	1 starch
Wild, cooked	½ cup	1	1 starch
Rice cakes, all flavors			
4" across	2 cakes	1	1 starch
Mini	½ oz	1	1 starch
Rye flour	3 Tbsp	1	1 starch
Soybean flour	½ cup	1	1 starch, 2 med. fat meat

Food	Quantity	Carbohydrate Choices	Exchanges
Low-fat	½ cup	1	1 starch, 3 lean meat
Tabouli	¼ cup	1½	1½ starch, 1 fat
Tempeh	½ cup	1	1 starch, 2 med. fat meat
Wheat berries, cooked	⅔ cup	1	1 starch
Wheat bran, toasted	⅓ cup	1	1 starch
Wheat germ, toasted	¼ cup	1	1 starch, 1 very lean meat
Vegetables with braised tofu	2 cups	1	1 starch, 1 veg, 1 med. fat meat, 2 fat
Vegetarian egg rolls with sweet and sour sauce	3 mini	1½	1½ starch, 1 veg

Milk

Goat milk	1 cup	1	1 milk, 1½ fat
Kefir	1 cup	1	1 milk, 1½ fat
Soy milk; *see also* Meat Substitutes below			
Regular	1 cup	1½	1½ milk, 1 fat
Light	1 cup	1	1 milk
Yogurt, nonfat plain	6 oz	1	1 milk
Yogurt, fruit-flavored, sweetened with a sugar substitute	8 oz	1	1 milk

Vegetable; *see also* Vegetable List

Bamboo shoots, cooked	½ cup	0	1 veg
Carrot juice	¼ cup	0	1 veg
Seaweed, cooked	½ cup	0	1 veg
Sprouts (alfalfa, bean, mung, soy)	1 cup raw or ¾ cup cooked	0	1 veg
Water chestnuts, canned	6 whole	0	1 veg

Meat Substitutes

Beans, dried, cooked			
Black beans (turtle beans)	1 cup	2	2 starch, 1 very lean meat
Broad beans (fava beans)	⅔ cup	2	2 starch, 1 very lean meat
Calico beans	1 cup	2	2 starch, 1 very lean meat

Food	Quantity	Carbohydrate Choices	Exchanges
Garbanzo beans (chickpeas)	⅔ cup	2	2 starch, 1 very lean meat
Kidney beans	1 cup	2	2 starch, 1 very lean meat
Lima beans	1 cup	2	2 starch, 1 very lean meat
Mung beans	1 cup	2	2 starch, 1 very lean meat
Navy beans	⅔ cup	2	2 starch, 1 very lean meat
Pinto beans	⅔ cup	2	2 starch, 1 very lean meat

Cheese; *see* Meat and Meat Substitutes List

La Loma® products

Food	Quantity	Carbohydrate Choices	Exchanges
Big franks, canned	1 frank	0	2 lean meat
Chicken, fried, frozen	1 piece (2 oz)	0	2 med. fat meat, 1 fat
Corn dogs, frozen	1 corn dog	1	1 starch, 2 med. fat meat
Griddle steak, frozen	1 steak (2 oz)	0	2 lean meat
Nuteena, canned	1 slice (½" thick)	0	1 med. fat meat, 2 fat
Savory meatballs, frozen	7 meatballs	0	1 veg, 3 lean meat
Swiss steak, canned	1 piece	0	1 veg, 2 med. fat meat
Vege-burger, canned	½ cup	0	3 lean meat
Lentils	1 cup	2	2 starch, 1 lean meat

Morningstar Farms® products

Food	Quantity	Carbohydrate Choices	Exchanges
Breakfast links, frozen	2 links	0	1 med. fat meat
Breakfast patty, frozen	1 patty	0	1 high fat meat
Scramblers, frozen	¼ cup	0	1 lean meat
Natto	½ cup	1	1 starch, 2 med. fat meat

Natural Touch® products

Food	Quantity	Carbohydrate Choices	Exchanges
Lentil rice loaf, frozen	2½" slice	0	1 med. fat meat, 1 fat
Vegetarian chili, canned	⅔ cup	1	1 starch, 2 med. fat meat

Food	Quantity	Carbohydrate Choices	Exchanges
Nuts			
Almonds	¼ cup (1 oz)	0	1 med. fat meat, 2 fat
Brazil nuts	¼ cup (1 oz)	0	1 high fat meat, 2 fat
Butternuts	¼ cup (1 oz)	0	1 med. fat meat, 2 fat
Peanut butter	1 Tbsp	0	1 high fat meat, 1 fat or 1 med. fat meat, 2 fat
Peanuts, roasted	¼ cup (1 oz)	0	1 med. fat meat, 2 fat
Pecans	¼ cup (1 oz)	0	1 med. fat meat, 2 fat
Pignolias, pine nuts	2 Tbsp	0	1 med. fat meat, 2 fat
Pistachio	47 nuts (1 oz)	0	1 med. fat meat, 2 fat
Walnuts	16–20 halves (1 oz)	0	1 med. fat meat, 2 fat
Peas, dried, cooked			
Black-eyed peas (cowpeas)	1 cup	2	2 starch, 1 lean meat
Split peas	⅔ cup	2	2 starch, 1 lean meat
Seeds			
Pumpkin or squash	¼ cup	0	1 med. fat meat, 2 fat
Sesame	¼ cup	0	1 med. fat meat, 2 fat
Sunflower	¼ cup	0	1 med. fat meat, 2 fat
Sunflowers with hulls	½ cup	0	1 med. fat meat, 2 fat
Soybeans, cooked	½ cup	½	½ starch, 1 med. fat meat
Soybean flour	½ cup	1	1 starch, 2 med. fat meat
Low-fat	½ cup	1	1 starch, 3 lean meat
Soy grits, raw	2 Tbsp	0	1 lean meat
Soy milk, fortified	1 cup	0	1½ other carb, 1 med. fat meat

Food	Quantity	Carbohydrate Choices	Exchanges
Tempeh	¼ cup	0	1 med. fat meat
	½ cup	1	1 starch, 2 med. fat meat
Tofu	½ cup	0	1 med. fat meat
Tofu hot dog	1 hot dog	0	1 med. fat meat
Vegetable protein, textured	¾ oz	½	½ starch, 1 lean meat
Worthington Foods® products			
Bolono, frozen	2 slices	0	1 lean meat
Chicken, frozen	2 slices	0	1 med. fat meat, 1 fat
Chili, canned	⅔ cup	1	1 starch, 1 med. fat meat, 1 fat
Choplets, canned	2 slices	0	2 lean meat
Corned beef, frozen	4 slices	½	½ starch, 1 med. fat meat
Country stew	9½ oz can	1	1 starch, 1 veg, 1 med. fat meat, 1 fat
Cutlets, canned	1½ slices	0	2 lean meat
Dinner roast, frozen	2 slices (3 oz)	0	1 high fat meat
Non-meat balls, canned	3 pieces	0	1 high fat meat
Prime stakes	1 piece	½	½ starch, 1 med. fat meat, 1 fat
Prosage links, frozen	2 links	0	1 high fat meat
Salami, meatless, frozen	2 slices	½	½ starch, 1 lean meat
Smoked beef, frozen	3 slices	½	½ starch, 1 med. fat meat
Smoked turkey, frozen	4 slices	0	2 lean meat
Tuno, frozen	2 oz	0	1 high fat meat
Turkee slices, canned	2 slices	0	1 med. fat meat, 1 fat
Vegetable skallops, canned	½ cup	0	2 lean meat
Vegetarian beef or chicken pie, frozen	1 pie	3	3 starch, 4 fat
Vegetarian burger, canned	½ cup	½	½ starch, 2 lean meat

Food	Quantity	Carbohydrate Choices	Exchanges
Vegetarian egg roll	1 large	1	1 starch, 1 veg, 1 fat
Wham, frozen	3 slices	0	2 med. fat meat
Fat			
Almond paste	2 tsp	0	1 fat
Bacon, simulated meat product	2 strips	0	1 fat
Lecithin	2 tsp	0	1 fat
Tahini paste	2 tsp	0	1 fat
Tofu cream cheese	1 Tbsp	0	1 fat
Free Foods			
Carob powder	1 Tbsp	0	free
Sprouts	½ cup	0	free

WORD LIST

Almond butter: A spreadable paste made from ground, toasted almonds.

Amaranth: A grain originally used by the ancient Aztecs, now often used combined with other grains. The seeds are yellowish brown and tiny.

Brewer's yeast: A savory, powdered flavoring used as a supplement in cooking. It does not rise like regular yeast.

Buckwheat: A bushlike plant. Buckwheat seeds are called groats, coarse ground groats are called grits, and finely ground groats are buckwheat flour.

Carob powder: A mildly sweet powder make by grinding the pods of the tropical carob tree. It is often used as a chocolate substitute because it tastes like cocoa.

Falafel: Patties made from coarse-ground wheat germ, garbanzo beans, fava beans, and spices, then lightly fried in oil.

Hummus: A spread made from pureed garbanzo beans (chickpeas), tahini, lemon juice, olive oil, and garlic.

Kasha: Buckwheat groats served as a cooked cereal or as a potato substitute.

Kefir: A cultured dairy product similar to milk.

Lecithin: Extracted from soybeans and used as a dietary supplement.

Legumes: Dried beans (kidney, garbanzo, navy, pinto, lima), peanuts, black-eyed peas, and lentils.

Meat analogs:	Foods made of vegetable protein that duplicate the flavor, texture, and appearance of meat.
Millet:	A tiny, round, yellowish grain widely used in Asia and Africa. Often served as a simple grain dish tossed with chopped onions and herbs.
Miso:	A rich, salty condiment made by combining soybeans, salt, a mold culture, and sometimes a grain such as rice; the mixture is then aged. Used to flavor soups, sauces, dressings, and marinades, and to make pâtes.
Natto:	Fermented, cooked soybean with a sticky, viscous coating and a cheesy texture.
Soybean:	A high-protein, high-fat bean used to make a variety of products such as tofu, tempeh, tamari, miso, soymilk, and textured vegetable protein.
Soymeat:	Spun soy protein products. The cheeselike curd from soybeans is mechanically manipulated to obtain a meatlike texture.
Tabouli:	A Middle Eastern salad made from bulgur and flavored with lemon and mint.
Tahini:	Sesame seed paste.
Tempeh:	Whole soybeans, usually mixed with another grain such as rice or millet, that are fermented and pressed into a solid cake. It can be marinated and grilled or baked in sauces.
Textured vegetable protein (TVP):	A name for textured soy protein, which is made from soy flour. Available in granules or chunks, this product is sometimes flavored to taste like meat and is used in place of ground beef in recipes.
Tofu:	Soft, unripened cheeselike curd made from soybeans.

CHAPTER 19

Asian Food Exchanges

Interesting spices and healthful ingredients make cuisines of Southeast Asia—Chinese, Japanese, and Thai—very popular among American diners. These cuisines share much in common, such as cooking methods, but they have subtle differences that make each a distinct dining experience.

Asian cuisines offer many selections that fit easily into a healthy diet. Cooking methods tend to be low fat, such as steaming, boiling, or stir-frying in a small amount of hot oil. Milk and cheese are rarely used, and only small portions of meat or seafood are used.

Traditional Asian eating utensils are chopsticks made of bamboo, wood, plastic, ivory or silver; these are accompanied by a porcelain spoon used for soup. Although chopsticks may be difficult to use at first, they can be mastered quickly with practice. A good way to learn is to pick up and hold peanuts, one at a time! It is considered bad manners to eat rice with the bowl resting on the table; instead, it should be raised to the mouth. All in all, new tastes and long-standing traditions can add up to a remarkable dining experience.

Chinese

There are four schools of Chinese cooking: Peking, characterized by the use of garlic, leeks, scallions, noodles, and dumplings; Shanghai, specializing in "red-cooking," a form of braising with large amounts of soy sauce and sugar; Szechwan and Hunan, famous for the liberal use of chile peppers and hot pepper sauces in spicy and somewhat greasy dishes; and Cantonese, the least greasy of all the regional styles, using fish, seafood, and vegetables. A Cantonese specialty is dim sum, which are dumplings stuffed with pork, shrimp, beef, sweet paste, or preserves; they are steamed or deep-fried and often served at brunch.

As you look for healthy Chinese foods, look for dishes cooked by the stir-fry method, such as chicken with broccoli or shrimp with Chinese vegetables, or by steaming, such as dim sum. Avoid meats that are deep-fried and then stir-fried, such as Peking chicken or crispy shrimp.

Good Choices	**Go Easy**
Hot-and-sour shrimp	Fried noodles
Wonton soup	Egg foo yung
Steamed dumplings	Crispy or batter-coated foods
Chicken chow mein	Egg rolls
Chicken and beef chop suey	Fried wontons
Chicken or vegetable lo mein	Sweet and sour chicken
Chicken or beef teriyaki	Cashew chicken
Moo shu shrimp or chicken	Barbecued spare ribs
Stir-fried meat with vegetables	Beef or pork fried rice
Steamed rice	
Lobster, hoisin, black bean, and plum sauces	
Fortune cookies	

Japanese

Japanese main dishes use a wide variety of vegetables, along with fish or small amounts of meat. They are seasoned with soy sauce and/or miso sauce, a soybean product. Glazes and sauces are typically made with low-fat ingredients: broth, soy sauce, rice wine, or sake. White rice is a staple, and a variety of fresh fruit is eaten. Simple cakes and cookies made of sugar and rice flour are also popular and contain little or no fat, although desserts are not usually part of a meal.

Most Japanese cuisine, with its emphasis on fresh fruits and vegetables and its low-fat cooking methods, fits easily into a healthy lifestyle. The exception is tempura (deep-fried fish, shellfish, or vegetables), one of the few Japanese cooking techniques in which fat is used. If you're trying to limit your sodium intake, be aware that the basis for much of the flavor in Japanese food is soy sauce (shoyu), which is high in salt.

Good Choices	Go Easy
Nabemono (boiled) or yaki-mono (broiled) dishes	Agemono
	Chicken katsu
Combinations of grilled meats or seafood and vegetables	Fried tofu
	Sukiyaki
Kayaku goban	Tempura
Miso and bean soups	Tonkatsu
Sashimi or sushi	Yakitori
Shabu shabu	Yosenabe
Shumai	
Soba or udon noodles	
Steamed rice	

Thai

Like other Asian cuisines, Thai meals use rice as the staple, accompanied by dishes that incorporate vegetables and small portions of beef, pork, poultry, and seafood. However, the flavoring of Thai food is not as dependent on soy sauce as other Asian cuisines. Instead, hot pepper sauce or crushed dried chiles, Thai spices, curry, and hot sauces add spice and "fire" to foods. Look for stir-fried, steamed, sautéed, boiled, marinated, grilled, and barbecued items on the menu. Be careful of foods fried in lard or prepared with coconut milk or cream.

Good Choices	Go Easy
Hang mung poo	Curries and soups based on coconut milk
Hot and sour soup	
Po tak	Crispy or deep-fried Thai rolls or tofu
Stir-fried noodles and sprouts	
Sautéed ginger beef or chicken	Crispy fried rice
	Coconut ice cream or puddings
	Peanut sauces

Sample Chinese Meal

Menu	**Exchanges**
Wonton soup, 1 cup	1 starch, 1 fat
Yu hsiang chicken, 1½ cups	1 veg, 2 med. fat meat
Beef with broccoli and black mushroom, 1 cup	1 veg, 2 med. fat meat
Steamed white rice, ⅔ cup	2 starch
Fortune cookie, 2 cookies	1 starch or 1 other carb

Meal Total

Exchanges:	4 starch (or 3 starch and 1 other carb), 2 veg, 4 med. fat meat, 1 fat
Calories:	700
Carbohydrate:	70 grams (40%)
Protein:	45 grams (25%)
Fat:	30 grams (35%)

Sample Japanese Meal

Menu	**Exchanges**
Su-udon soup, 1 cup	1 starch, 1 fat
Donburi, oyako, 1½ cup	3 starch, 1 veg, 1 med. fat meat
Teriyaki salmon, 4 oz	4 lean meat
Steamed rice, ⅓ cup	1 starch

Meal Total

Exchanges:	5 starch, 1 veg, 4 lean meat, 1 med. fat meat, 1 fat
Calories:	750
Carbohydrate:	80 grams (43%)
Protein:	45 grams (24%)
Fat:	28 grams (33%)

Sample Thai Meal

Menu	**Exchanges**
Tom yum koong soup, 1 cup	1 starch
Tai chicken, 1 cup	1 veg, 2 lean meat, 1 fat
Poy sian, 1 cup	1 veg, 2 lean meat, 1 fat
Steamed rice, 1 cup	3 starch
Hot tea	free

Meal Total	
Exchanges:	4 starch, 2 veg, 4 lean meat, 2 fat
Calories:	700
Carbohydrate:	70 grams (41%)
Protein:	45 grams (26%)
Fat:	25 grams (33%)

ASIAN FOOD LIST

Food	Quantity	Carbohydrate Choices	Exchanges
Starch			
Adzuki beans, cooked	⅓ cup	1	1 starch
Almond cookie	2 medium	1	1 starch or 1 other carb
Arrowroot starch	2 Tbsp	1	1 starch
Bow (Chinese steamed dough)	1 small or ⅔ medium	1	1 starch
Cellophane noodles, cooked	¾ cup	1	1 starch
Chinese noodles	⅓ cup	1	1 starch
Chow mein noodles	½ cup	1	1 starch, 1 fat
Chestnuts	4 large or 6 small	1	1 starch
Cornstarch	2 Tbsp	1	1 starch
Congee rice soup	¾ cup	1	1 starch
Egg roll wrapper	2 wrappers	1	1 starch
Fortune cookie	2 cookies	1	1 starch or 1 other carb
Fried rice	⅓ cup	1	1 starch, 1 fat
	1 cup	3	3 starch, 3 fat
Ginkgo seeds	½ cup	1	1 starch
Glutinous rice (Sticky rice)	⅓ cup	1	1 starch
Lotus root	10 slices	1	1 starch
Miso	3 Tbsp	1	1 starch
	½ cup	2½	2½ starch, 1 med. fat meat
Mung beans, cooked	⅓ cup	1	1 starch
Mung bean noodles	¾ cup	1	1 starch
Poi (taro), cooked	⅓ cup	1	1 starch
Red beans, cooked	⅓ cup	1	1 starch
Rice, cooked, loosely packed	⅓ cup	1	1 starch
Rice noodles, vermicelli, cooked	½ cup	1	1 starch
Rice soup	¾ cup	1	1 starch
Soba noodles	½ cup	1	1 starch
Su-udon soup	1 cup	1	1 starch, 1 fat
Tom yum koong soup	1 cup	1	1 starch

Food	Quantity	Carbohydrate Choices	Exchanges
Udon noodles	½ cup	1	1 starch
Wonton wrappers, 3" x 3"	4 wrappers	1	1 starch
Wonton, fried	3 medium	1	1 starch, 3 fat
Wheat fritters	1 medium	1	1 starch
Yard-long beans, pods, and seeds	1 cup	1	1 starch
Fruit			
Apple pear (Asian pear)	1 medium	1	1 fruit
Carambola	1½ medium	1	1 fruit
Dried salted apricots	6 halves	1	1 fruit
Guava	1 medium	1	1 fruit
Kumquats	5 medium	1	1 fruit
Longans	30 medium	1	1 fruit
Canned	¾ cup	1	1 fruit
Loquat	5–6 fruits	1	1 fruit
Lychees, fresh or dried	10 medium	1	1 fruit
Canned	½ cup	1	1 fruit
Mango	½ medium	1	1 fruit
Papaya	½ fruit	1	1 fruit
Persimmon, Japanese	½ medium	1	1 fruit
Pomelo	¾ cup	1	1 fruit
Red dates	6 medium	1	1 fruit
Milk			
Coconut milk	1 cup	½	½ milk, 7 fat
Light	1 cup	½	½ milk, 3 fat
Soy milk	1 cup	1½	1½ milk, 1 fat
Vegetable			
Arrowroot	1 (2" across)	0	1 veg
Bamboo shoots, canned	½ cup	0	1 veg
Bean sprouts	1 cup raw or ¾ cup cooked	0	1 veg
Bitter melon	½ cup	0	1 veg
Bok choy, cooked	1 cup	0	1 veg
Button or straw mushrooms	½ cup	0	1 veg
Chayote	½ cup	0	1 veg
Chinese cabbage	2 cups raw or 1 cup cooked	0	1 veg

Food	Quantity	Carbohydrate Choices	Exchanges
Chinese spinach, cooked	½ cup	0	1 veg
Corn, baby, canned	½ cup	0	1 veg
Daikon (Chinese radish)	1 cup	0	1 veg
Fuzzy melon	½ cup	0	1 veg
Ginger root	¼ cup	0	1 veg
Kohlrabi	⅔ cup	0	1 veg
Leeks (Chinese onion)	½ cup or 2 medium	0	1 veg
Miso	1 Tbsp	0	1 veg
Mushrooms, dried, black	¼ cup	0	1 veg
Mustard leaves	½ cup	0	1 veg
Nori	1 small sheet	0	1 veg
Peas (snow, sugar, sweet, or peapods)	½ cup	0	1 veg
Seaweed laver, soaked	½ cup	0	1 veg
Seahair, soaked	½ cup	0	1 veg
Taro root	¼ cup	0	1 veg

Meat/Meat Substitutes

Food	Quantity	Carbohydrate Choices	Exchanges
Abalone	1 oz	0	1 lean meat
Chicken wings	1 wing	0	1 lean meat
Chinese sausage	½ sausage (1 oz)	0	1 high fat meat
Duck egg, preserved	1 egg	0	1 high fat meat
Duck feet	3 medium	0	1 med. fat meat
Eel	1 oz	0	1 high fat meat
Fish maw	2 oz	0	1 med. fat meat
Horse beans (broad beans)	⅔ cup	2	2 starch, 1 lean meat
Octopus	2 oz	0	1 lean meat
Oxtail	1 oz	0	1 med. fat meat
Pork feet	2 oz	0	1 high fat meat
Poy sian	1 cup	0	1 veg, 2 lean meat, 1 fat
Red mung beans	⅔ cup	2	2 starch, 1 lean meat
Scallops, dried	1 large	0	1 lean meat
Shrimp, dried	10 shrimp (½ oz)	0	1 lean meat
Squid	1 oz	0	1 very lean meat
Tofu	½ cup (4 oz)	0	1 med. fat meat

Food	Quantity	Carbohydrate Choices	Exchanges
Fat			
Chicken fat or pork fat	1 tsp	0	1 fat
Coconut milk	2 Tbsp	0	1 fat
Light	¼ cup	0	1 fat
Coconut, grated	2 Tbsp	0	1 fat
Macadamia nuts	3 medium	0	1 fat
Pork, cured	1" cube	0	1 fat
Sesame or peanut oil	1 tsp	0	1 fat
Sesame paste	2 tsp	0	1 fat
Sesame seeds	1 Tbsp	0	1 fat
Watermelon seeds	⅓ oz	0	1 fat
Free Foods			
Coriander	–	0	free
Curry	–	0	free
Dipping sauce	2 Tbsp	0	free
Fish sauce	–	0	free
Fortune cookie	1 cookie	0	free
	2 cookies	1	1 other carb
Garlic	–	0	free
Ginger	–	0	free
Green onion	–	0	free
Hot mustard	–	0	free
Miso dressing	2 Tbsp	0	free
Soy sauce (tamari)	–	0	free
Sweet and sour sauce	1 Tbsp	0	free
Star anise	–	0	free
Combination Foods			
Beef and vegetables	2 cups	2	2 starch, 1 veg, 2 med. fat meat
Cashew nut chicken	1 cup	1	1 starch, 2 med. fat meat, 4 fat
Chicken and vegetables	2 cups	2	2 starch, 1 veg, 2 lean meat
Chinese broccoli with beef or pork	1 cup	1	1 starch, 3 med. fat meat, 2–3 fat

Food	Quantity	Carbohydrate Choices	Exchanges
Chop suey	2 cups	2	2 starch, 3–4 med. fat meat, 1–2 fat
Chow luny aas	¾ cup	0	3 med. fat meat, 1 fat
Chow mein (beef, pork, or chicken)	2 cups	2	2 starch, 1 veg, 2–3 med. fat meat, 1–2 fat
Crispy shrimp	1 cup	2	2 starch, 3 med. fat meat, 4–5 fat
Dim sum			
Gow-Gee	3 pieces	1	1 starch, 1 med. fat meat
Har-Gow	3 pieces	½	½ starch, ½ med. fat meat
Siu-Mai	2 pieces	½	½ starch, 1 med. fat meat
War-Tip	2 pieces	½	½ starch, 1 med. fat meat
Donburi, oyako	1½ cups	3	3 starch, 1 veg, 1 med. fat meat
Egg drop soup	1 cup	0	½ med. fat meat
Egg flower soup	2 cups	0	1 med. fat meat
Egg foo yung	1 medium patty	0	1 veg, 2 med. fat meat, 2 fat
Egg foo yung sauce	¼ cup	0	1 veg
Egg roll (chicken, pork, or shrimp)	1 small	1	1 starch, 1 med. fat meat, 2 fat
Fried rice (rice, meat, eggs, and onion)	1 cup	2	2 starch, 1 med. fat meat, 2 fat
Fung gawn aar	1 cup	0	3 med. fat meat, 2 fat
Hot and sour soup	1 cup	0	1 veg, 1 med. fat meat
Mock duck	1 cup	1	1 starch, 2 lean meat
Moo goo gai pan	2 cups	1	1 starch, 1 veg, 2–3 med. fat meat, 0–1 fat

Food	Quantity	Carbohydrate Choices	Exchanges
Moo shi shrimp	2 pancakes with 1 cup filling	1	1 starch, 2 veg, 2 med. fat meat, 1 fat
Mum yee mein	1 cup	2	2 starch, 2 med. fat meat, 1 fat
Peking ravioli, steamed	2 medium	1	1 starch, 1 med. fat meat, 1 fat
Pepper steak	1 cup	1	1 starch, 3 med. fat meat, 1 veg
Ramaki	2 pieces	0	1 med. fat meat, 1 fat
Rice soup	¾ cup	1	1 starch
Shiu mi	2 pieces	½	½ starch, ½ fat
Shrimp and vegetables	2 cups	2	2 starch, 1 veg, 2 lean meat
Shrimp with broccoli and mushrooms	1 cup	0	1 veg, 2 med. fat meat, 1 fat
Siumoni soup	1 cup	0	1 veg
Snow pea shrimp or chicken	1 cup	1	1 starch, 2–3 med. fat meat, 2 fat
Sukiyaki	1½ cup	0	3 med. fat meat, 1 fat
Sweet and sour pork or shrimp	1 cup	4	4 starch, 2 med. fat meat, 1–2 fat
Tai chicken	1 cup	0	1 veg, 2 lean meat, 1 fat
Vegetable lo mein noodles	1½ cup	3	3 starch, 1 veg, 1 fat
Wonton, boiled	4 wonton	1	1 starch, 1 med. fat meat, 1 fat
Wonton soup	2 wonton and 1 cup broth	1	1 starch, 1 fat
Yaki-udon soup	1 cup	0	1 veg, 1 fat
Yu hsiang chicken	1 cup with ⅓ cup rice	1	1 starch, 1 veg, 2 med. fat meat

WORD LIST

Abalone:	A delicate, bland-tasting mollusk often used in main dishes.
Adzuki beans:	A small brownish bean used frequently in Japanese cooking and often served mixed with brown rice or other grains.
Agemono:	Japanese word meaning "deep-fried things."
Bean curd:	Smooth, creamy, custardlike product, made from pureed soybeans that are formed into blocks. Known as "tofu" in the United States.
Bean sprouts:	Tiny white bean shoots with pale green hoods.
Bitter melon (balsam pear):	Cucumber-like vegetable with a bumpy green surface and bitter flavor.
Black beans, fermented:	A tangy spice used in Chinese cooking to darken sauces or as a main ingredient.
Black mushrooms:	Dried fungi used extensively in Chinese cooking. Also known as Chinese or winter mushrooms.
Bok choy:	Vegetable with broad white or greenish-white stalks and loose, dark-green leaves. Also known as Chinese chard or white mustard cabbage.
Carambola (star fruit):	Glossy, yellow pods marked with five longitudinal ribs that form a star shape when the fruit is sliced.
Cellophane noodles:	Hard, opaque, fine, white noodles made from ground mung beans.
Chili paste:	Condiment made with mashed chile peppers, vinegar, and garlic.
Chow luny aas:	Lobster tails in garlic sauce.
Coconut milk:	A creamy liquid extracted from grating fresh coconut meat (not the liquid inside the coconut).
Congee:	Chinese soupy rice gruel.
Coriander:	Spice with a pungent, musky flavor. Its fresh, leafy version is known as cilantro or Chinese parsley.
Dim sum:	Steamed or fried dumplings stuffed with meat, seafood, and/or vegetables, sweet paste, or preserves.
Donburi:	Dish served on a bed of rice with special sauce.
Duck feet:	Duck feet braised in soy sauce, sugar, wine, salt, monosodium glutamate, and spices.
Duck eggs, preserved:	Duck eggs soaked in brine for thirty to forty days.
Duck sauce:	Sauce made by blending plums, apricots, vinegar, and sugar. Also known as plum sauce.
Egg roll:	Minced or shredded meat and/or seafood and vegetables wrapped in egg roll wrapper and deep-fried.
Fish maw:	Dried and deep-fried stomach lining of fish.

Fish sauce:	A sauce made by fermenting small, salted fish in wooden casks for several months and draining the liquid.
Fung gawn aar:	Shrimp, chicken liver, and mushrooms in chicken broth.
Ginkgo nuts or seeds:	Small fruit of Ginkgo tree with tough, beige-colored shells and ivory-colored nuts.
Glutinous rice:	A short-grained, pearl white rice that becomes sticky and translucent when cooked. Also known as sweet or sticky rice.
Hoisin sauce:	Sauce made from fermented mashed soybeans, salt, sugar, and garlic. Also known as Chinese barbecue sauce.
Hang mung poo:	Spicy steamed mussels.
Katsuo:	A dried bonita (fish belonging to the mackerel family). A basic ingredient of Japanese stock.
Kohlrabi:	A member of the cabbage family with a delicate, turnip-like taste. Bulbs may be steamed or eaten raw.
Kayaku goban:	Japanese dish consisting of vegetables and rice.
Longan:	A small, round fruit with a smooth, brown skin and clear pulp. Fresh longans come in clusters, but the canned product is more common.
Loquat:	A small, round fruit with yellow-orange skin and pale yellow to orange flesh with black seeds. The flavor is like a blend of banana and pineapple.
Lotus root:	Tuberous stem of the water lily.
Lychee (lichee, litchi):	A small, delicate, juicy, round fruit used as dessert, as a garnish, or in sweet and sour dishes.
Miso:	A rich, salty condiment made by combining soybeans, salt, a mold culture, and sometimes a grain such as rice; the mixture is then aged. Used to flavor soups, sauces, dressings, and marinades, and to make pâtes.
Mock duck:	Vegetarian mixed dish that commonly consists of wheat gluten cooked with vegetables.
Mum yee mein:	Braised noodles, chicken breast, mushrooms, chestnuts, and Chinese peas.
Nori:	A sea vegetable sold in flat, dried sheets. Often used to make sushi or nori rolls.
Oyako:	Sautéed chicken, eggs, and onions.
Persimmon:	A bright orange fruit with a shiny skin that is removed before eating. Known as the "apple of the Orient."
Po tak:	Hot and sour seafood in lemon juice.
Poi:	A thick paste with a starchy, mild taste made from the ground, cooked roots of the taro plant.
Pomelo:	A citrus fruit that is green, yellow, or pink in color. Also known as Chinese grapefruit.
Ramaki:	Chicken livers and water chestnuts wrapped in bacon.

Rice noodles: Very thin strands of translucent noodles often sold in coiled nests.

Rice vermicelli: Thin, white noodles made from rice flour, often used as an alternative to rice.

Sashimi: Sliced, raw fish.

Shabu shabu: A dish of sliced beef and vegetables that is cooked and served at the table with noodles and a special sauce.

Shiu mi: Chopped chestnuts, chives, and pork wrapped in thin noodles.

Shumai: Steamed dumplings.

Soba noodles: Japanese noodles made from buckwheat

Spring roll wrapper: Thin sheets made from rice flour; larger than wonton wrappers.

Suimono soup: Clear broth.

Sukiyaki: A meat and vegetable dinner.

Sushi: Rice mixed with rice vinegar, often served with sliced raw fish (sashimi).

Szechwan: A style of Chinese cooking characterized by use of fiery pepper sauces.

Tamari: Soy sauce made in the traditional Asian way, which requires long periods of fermentation and aging.

Taro: Starchy, tuberous, rough-textured brown root.

Tempura: Deep-fried fish, shellfish, or vegetables.

Teriyaki: A method of cooking using a sweet soy-seasoned glaze.

Tofu: Soft, unripened cheeselike curd made from soybeans.

Tonkatsu: Fried pork.

Udon noodles: Flat whole wheat noodles used in Asian cooking.

Wonton: A steamed or fried wrapper filled with minced pork and/or shrimp.

Wonton wrappers: Thin, yellow sheets made of flour, egg, salt, and water.

Yakitori: Chicken teriyaki.

Yaki-udon soup: Buckwheat noodle soup with stir-fried vegetables.

Yard-long beans: Thin, flexible, tender beans that can grow to a length of up to eighteen inches.

Yu hsiang chicken: Strips of chicken stir-fried with bamboo shoots, water chestnuts, wood ears, lily buds, and Chinese cabbage.

CHAPTER 20

Exchanges Mexican Style

From simple snacks like chips and salsa to upscale restaurant meals, foods from Mexico and the American Southwest have a central place in our culinary melting pot. Using grains, beans, and chiles as staples, south-of-the-border dishes can add spice to your meals along with good nutrition. To fire up your food plan, try some of the dishes influenced by our neighbors to the south!

Beans—pinto beans, kidney beans, and black beans—are found in many Mexican dishes. Refried beans, a common menu item, are usually made from pinto beans. Whole-grain tortillas are served warm at almost every meal and come in two versions: the slightly coarse, light golden cornmeal variety and the softer white flour tortillas. Other common ingredients in Mexican foods are chicken, beef, eggs, and potatoes.

Southwestern cooking borrows heavily from Mexican cooking but has been influenced by Native American, Spanish, and American pioneer cooking as well. These cultures contributed ingredients such as corn, rice, squash, game, garlic, and onions. Cowboy culture also had a hand in southwestern cuisine, introducing cooking methods such as barbecuing and stewing. Cilantro, the fresh, citrusy green leaf of the coriander plant, makes an appearance in many dishes. Salsa (a sauce made of tomatoes and chiles) is the "salt and pepper" of the Southwest, but its popularity is no longer limited to that region.

Spices common in Mexican and southwestern cooking include garlic, cumin, chili powder (a blend of ground red chiles, oregano, cumin, and garlic) and chile peppers. The chile pepper is one of the world's most popular spices, and there are over one hundred varieties ranging from mild to fiery. In general, the smaller the pepper, the hotter it is. Although not recommended, the only beverage able to hold its own against the hottest chile pepper is tequila. Tequila is an alcohol distilled from the fermented juice of the maguey cactus plant, which thrives in the Mexican state of Jalisco.

The basic ingredients used in Mexican and southwestern cooking—corn, beans, tortillas, and tomatoes—are low in fat. However, extras like cheese and sour cream can boost the fat content of Mexican meals to much higher levels. Salt pork, bacon fat, and other animal fat drippings are also frequently used in Mexican cooking. Watch out for foods made with lard; this includes most refried beans, although lard-free versions are available in most supermarkets. Soft or baked tortillas are better choices than fried tortillas or deep-fried taco shells. When preparing Mexican foods yourself, omit saturated fats or substitute vegetable oil for

Good Choices

Arroz con pollo (remove the skin)

Bean, vegetable, chicken, or fish soft burritos

Beans or refried beans (without lard)

Black bean soup

Ceviche

Chicken enchiladas

Chicken, beef, or shrimp fajitas

Chicken, seafood, or bean enchiladas

Gazpacho soup

Hot sauce or chili sauce

Mexican rice

Plain yogurt and yogurt sauces

Red beans and rice

Salsa, salsa verde, or picante sauce

Shrimp or fish Veracruz

Soft chicken tacos

Tomato, onion, and avocado salad (with a squeeze of lemon juice)

Go Easy

Carne asada

Cheese

Chili con queso

Chile rellenos

Chimichangas

Chorizo

Fried dishes

Fried ice cream

Fried tamales

Guacamole

Huevos reales

Mole polo

Nachos

Refried beans (with lard)

Sopapillas

Sour cream

them. When you're planning to eat at a Mexican restaurant, use few or no fat choices at other times during the day. Also, choose what to eat and what to take home in a "doggie bag" or leave behind, if the full meal is too much for your meal plan.

Sample Mexican Meal

Menu	Exchanges
Black bean soup, 1 cup	2 starch
Chicken enchilada, 1 enchilada	2 starch, 2 med. fat meat, 1–2 fat
Beef taco, 1 taco	1 starch, 1 med. fat meat, 1 fat
Spanish rice, ½ cup	1 starch, 1 veg

Meal Total

Exchanges:	6 starch, 1 veg, 3 med. fat meat, 2–3 fat
Calories:	800
Carbohydrate:	95 grams (46%)
Protein:	40 grams (20%)
Fat:	30 grams (34%)

MEXICAN FOOD LIST

Food	Quantity	Carbohydrate Choices	Exchanges
Starch			
Amaranth, cooked	½ cup	1	1 starch
Beans			
Black, boiled or canned	½ cup	1	1 starch
Pinto or kidney, boiled or canned	⅓ cup	1	1 starch
	1 cup	2	2 starch, 1 very lean meat
Refried	⅓ cup	1	1 starch, 1 fat
Black bean soup	1 cup	2	2 starch
Bolillo	1½" piece	1	1 starch
Breadfruit	2 wedges (2"x1")	1	1 starch
Cassava	½ cup	1	1 starch
Corn chips	1 cup (1 oz)	1	1 starch, 2 fat
Corn bread	2" square	1	1 starch, 1 fat
Hard roll			
3" across	1 roll	1	1 starch
6" across	⅓ roll	1	1 starch
Hominy	½ cup	1	1 starch
"Hops" bread	1 small	1	1 starch
Jicama	1 cup	1	1 starch
Malanga	⅓ cup	1	1 starch
Masa harina	2 Tbsp	1	1 starch
Plantain, mature, cooked	⅓ large	1	1 starch
Spanish rice	⅓ cup	1	1 starch, 1 fat
Taco shell, 6" across	2 shells	1	1 starch, 1 fat
Tortillas			
Corn, 6" across	1 tortilla	1	1 starch
Flour, 7–8" across	1 tortilla	1	1 starch
Flour, 12" across	1 tortilla	2	2 starch
Tortilla chips, fried	6–12 chips (1 oz)	1	1 starch, 2 fat
Vermicelli	½ cup	1	1 starch
Yam, white	½ cup	1	1 starch
Yautia	1 small	1	1 starch
Boiled	⅓ cup		

Food	Quantity	Carbohydrate Choices	Exchanges
Fruit			
Apple banana	½ medium	1	1 fruit
Cactus fruit	1 medium	1	1 fru t
Cherimoya	½ small	1	1 fruit
Coco plum	1 medium	1	1 fruit
Guava	1 medium	1	1 fruit
Guava nectar	½ cup	1	1 fruit
Mamey	½ medium	1	1 fruit
Mango	½ small	1	1 fruit
Papaya	1 cup cubes	1	1 fruit
Sapota (Custard apple)	1 small	1	1 fruit
Other Carbohydrates			
Flan (Mexican custard)	1 cup	3	3 other carb, 3 fat
Pan dulce (sweet bread)	1 (4½" across)	4	4 other carb, 1 fat
Sopa (sweet Spanish bread soup)	1 cup	4	4 other carb, 2 fat
Vegetable			
Calabazita, cooked	½ cup	0	1 veg
Chayote	½ cup	0	1 veg
Cactus leaves (Nopales)	½ cup	0	1 veg
Gazpacho	½ cup	0	1 veg
Jalapeno peppers	4 peppers	0	1 veg
Jicama	½ cup	0	1 veg
Okra	½ cup	0	1 veg
Spanish sauce	½ cup	1	1 veg
Tomatoes, green	½ cup or 2 small	0	1 veg
Verdolaga (purslane)	½ cup	0	1 veg
Meat/Meat Substitutes			
Chorizo, beef or pork	1 oz	0	1 high fat meat, 1 fat
Goat meat	4 small cubes	0	1 med. fat meat
Queso (cheese) Jalisco, fresco, or Mexican	1 oz	0	1 med. fat meat
Skirt steak	1 oz	0	1 lean meat

Food	Quantity	Carbohydrate Choices	Exchanges
Fat			
Ackee	3 pieces	0	1 fat
Avocado	⅛ medium (4" across)	0	1 fat
Ghee	1 tsp	0	1 fat
Guacamole	2 Tbsp	0	1 fat
Sofrito	2 tsp	0	1 fat
Free Foods			
Chile peppers	–	0	free
Cilantro, fresh	–	0	free
Salsa	¼ cup	0	free
Taco sauce	–	0	free
Combination Foods			
Arroz con pollo	¾ cup	1	1 starch, 2 med. fat meat, 1 fat
Beef cubes in brown gravy (carne guisada)	1 cup	1	1 starch, 2 med. fat meat, 1 fat
Burrito de carne (meat with flour tortilla)			
7" across	1 burrito	2	2 starch, 2 med. fat meat, 1 fat (If deep-fried, add extra fat)
9" across	1 burrito	3	3 starch, 3 med. fat meat, 1 fat
Burrito de frijoles refritos (refried beans with flour tortilla)			
7" across	1 burrito	3	3 starch, 1 med. fat meat, 2 fat (If deep-fried, add 1 to 2 extra fat)
9" across	1 burrito	4	4 starch, 1½ med. fat meat, 2 fat
Chicken and yellow squash	¾ cup	0	2 lean meat, 1 veg, 2 fat

Food	Quantity	Carbohydrate Choices	Exchanges
Chili con carne			
With beans	1 cup	2	2 starch, 2 med. fat meat
Without beans	1 cup	½	½ starch, 3 med. fat meat
Chili rellenos	1 pepper (7" long)	2	2 starch, 1 veg, 2 med. fat meat, 3 fat
Chili verde (diced meat, green chile, rice or beans)	1 cup	1	1 starch, 1 veg, 3 med. fat meat, 2 fat
Chimichangas, all varieties	1 (6 oz)	3	3 starch, 2 med. fat meat, 2 fat
Corn fritters	1 (3" across)	1	1 starch, 2 med. fat meat, 1 fat
Enchiladas, beef or chicken (6" tortilla, meat, mozzarella cheese, red chili sauce)	1 enchilada	2	2 starch, 2 med. fat meat, 1–2 fat
Enchiladas, cheese (6" tortilla, mozzarella cheese, red chili sauce)	1 enchilada	2	2 starch, 1–2 med. fat meat, 3–4 fat
Enchirito with cheese, beef, and beans	1 medium	2	2 starch, 2 med. fat meat, 1 fat
Ensalada de aquacite	½ cup	0	1 veg, 3 fat
Fajitas (beef or chicken)	2 fajitas	4	4 starch, 3 med. fat meat, 2 fat
Flauta (rolled, filled, fried corn tortilla)	1 flauta	1	1 starch, 1 med. fat meat
Frijoles with cheese	1 cup	2	2 starch, 1 med. fat meat, 2 fat
Menudo	½ cup	0	1 lean meat
Mexican rice	½ cup	1	1 starch, 1 veg, 1 fat
Mexican squash with beef	½ cup	0	1 med. fat meat, 1 veg, 1 fat

Food	Quantity	Carbohydrate Choices	Exchanges
Nachos with cheese	6–8 nachos	2½	2½ starch, 1 high fat meat, 2 fat
Nachos with cheese, beans, and ground beef	6–8 nachos	3½	3½ starch, 2 med. fat meat, 3 fat
Picadillo	¾ cup	1	1 starch, 2 med. fat meat, 2 fat
Quesadillas (6" corn or 7" flour tortilla, green chiles, mozzarella cheese)	1 quesadilla	2	2 starch, 2 med. fat meat, 1 fat
Spanish rice	½ cup	1	1 starch, 1 veg
Taco (taco shell, meat, cheese, tomato, lettuce)			
Small (6–7")	1 taco	1	1 starch, 1 to 2 med. fat meat, 1 fat
Large	1 taco	3	3 starch, 3 med. fat meat, 3 fat
Taco, open (6–7" tortilla, ground beef, lettuce, chile sauce)	1 taco	1	1 starch, 3 med. fat meat, 1 veg
Taco salad (in fried tortilla shell, with sour cream, guacamole, and black olives)	1 large	3	4 starch, 1 vegetable, 3 med. fat meat, 5 fat
Tamales, beef (with sauce)	2 small or 1 large	2	2 starch, 1–2 med. fat meat, 2 fat
Tostada or tortilla with refried beans	1 small	2	2 starch, 2 fat
Tostada			
Beef	1 small	1	1 starch, 1 med. fat meat, 1 fat
Beef and cheese	1 large	1½	1½ starch, 2 med. fat meat, 1 fat
Beef, cheese, and beans	1 large	2	2 starch, 2 med. fat meat, 2 fat

Food	Quantity	Carbohydrate Choices	Exchanges
Beef, cheese, and beans with guacamole	1 large	2	2 starch, 2 med. fat meat, 3 fat
Vermicelli or rice with beef (fidelio con carne)	1 cup	2	2 starch, 2 med. fat meat, 1 fat

WORD LIST

Ackee:	Although the ackee is a fruit, it is usually cooked and served as a vegetable. When cooked its taste is similar to scrambled eggs.
Amaranth:	A grain originally used by the ancient Aztecs, now often used with other grains.
Apple banana:	Also called manzano or finger banana.
Arroz:	Rice.
Arroz con pollo:	Rice with chicken, tomatoes, and spices.
Atole:	Hot beverage made of milk or water, sugar, and corn-starch thickener. Vanilla, cinnamon, chocolate, or other flavors may be added.
Bolillo:	Similar to a French roll. May replace tortillas or be used to make a sandwich.
Burrito:	A soft flour tortilla filled with beans, ground beef, chicken, or cheese. It is rolled and covered with a sauce or deep-fried.
Cactus fruit:	Also known as a prickly pear fruit.
Café con leche:	Coffee with milk.
Calabacitas:	Mexican squash that is similar in size and shape to the cucumber and has light-green skin. Often simmered with onion and spices and/or combined with meat in a casserole dish.
Carne:	Meat.
Carne guisada:	Beef tips sautéed with chopped onions, green pepper, and chili peppers. Stewed tomatoes are added and the combination is simmered until tender.
Cassava:	Large, starchy root with a bitter odor that disappears after cooking. The starch derived from this root is used to make tapioca. Also called manioc or Yucca root.
Ceviche:	Marinated seafood.
Chayote:	Mexican squash that is light green, pear-shaped, and sometimes covered with tiny hairs.

Chirimoya:	A heart-shaped fruit with a rough, green outer skin. When ripened and chilled, the flesh has a sherbetlike texture. Also called sweet sop, sherbet fruit, or custard apple.
Chiles:	Refers to the chile pepper, of which there are over 100 varieties ranging in flavor from mild to sweet to pungent to red hot. Used fresh, canned, or dried, or as an ingredient in sauces or dishes.
Chili con carne:	Commonly referred to as chili. A hearty soup made with tomato, onions, peppers, kidney beans, spices, and beef.
Chili powder:	Blend of chiles, herbs, and spices.
Chile rellenos:	Green chile pepper filled with cheese and wrapped in a rich egg batter. Deep-fried and smothered in chili verde.
Chimichanga:	Flour tortilla filled and folded like a burrito, then deep-fried.
Chorizo:	A highly seasoned sausage of chopped beef or pork with sweet red peppers. Frequently fried and eaten in a taco, burrito, or tortilla mixed with scrambled eggs.
Cilantro:	The fresh leaves and stems of the coriander plant.
Enchilada:	Oil-blanched corn tortilla folded (or rolled) around a filling of beef or cheese. It can be covered with a sauce of chili con carne, tomato, cheese, or guacamole and garnished with chopped onions and grated cheese.
Enchirito:	Enchilada with meat, chiles, beans, and sauce.
Ensalada de aquacite:	Sliced avocado with tomato and lettuce.
Fajitas:	Chicken, beef, or shrimp sautéed with onions, peppers, tomatoes, and Mexican spices. Served in a skillet, with flour tortillas and salsa on the side.
Fidelio con carne:	Sautéed beef cubes combined with browned vermicelli, tomatoes, and spices.
Flan (Mexican custard):	A sweetened egg custard topped with caramelized sugar.
Flauta:	A rolled, filled, fried corn tortilla.
Frijoles:	Beans. Served in some form at nearly every meal in Mexico, they are frequently simmered until tender with onion, cilantro, chile pepper, diced tomatoes, and seasonings.
Frijoles cocidos:	Boiled beans.
Frijoles refritos:	Refried beans. Prepared by simmering beans with bacon, onion, garlic, whole tomatoes, cilantro, and herbs until soft, then mashing and frying them slowly. Chili powder may be added.
Ghee:	Butter that has been clarified or gently warmed over low heat until it browns lightly, giving it a distinct aroma. It is used as a flavoring or as a topping for rice and breads.

Guacamole:	Mashed avocado mixture sometimes seasoned with salsa, chopped chiles, and other seasonings.
Guava:	A sweet, juicy fruit containing many small seeds in the center. Its outer skin ranges in color from green to yellow, and its inner flesh ranges from white to salmon red.
Harina:	Flour.
Huevos reales:	Dessert made with egg yolks, sugar, sherry, cinnamon, pine nuts, and raisins.
Jícama:	A large, lumpy tuber with dull brown skin and a crisp, white, juicy flesh.
Maize:	Corn.
Malanga:	Large herb with a starchy, thick, tuberous, white, edible root.
Manteca:	Lard.
Masa harina:	Specially-prepared corn flour used to make corn tortillas, tamales, and nachos.
Menudo:	Tripe and hominy soup. A popular weekend breakfast dish.
Mexican rice:	White rice sautéed in a skillet with tomatoes, green peppers, onions, and seasonings.
Mole:	Sauce or gravy of dried red chiles, chocolate, chicken broth, cinnamon, sesame seeds, nuts, and other spices. Served on special occasions, this sauce is usually cooked with chicken or turkey and served with tortillas, beans, and rice.
Nachos:	Fried tortilla chips with cheese.
Nopales (cactus):	The leaves or pods of the prickly pear cactus, which are sliced in strips and cooked with onions and spices. They taste like crisp green beans.
Pan dulce:	Sweet bread or sweet rolls served at breakfast or as an afternoon or evening snack. Generally lower in fat and sugar than the American equivalent.
Pescado:	Fish.
Picadillo:	A type of beef has that is flavored with traditional Spanish ingredients of olives and raisins, as well as Caribbean tomatoes and hot chiles.
Picante:	The Mexican word for "hot and spicy."
Plantain:	A greenish banana with a rough, blemished skin which remains starchy even when fully ripe. Never eaten raw.
Quesadillas:	Tortillas filled with cheese and heated or fried until cheese melts. They are eaten with salsa, usually as snacks.
Queso fresco, blanco, or mexicano:	White, crumbly, Mexican cheese that is low in fat. Similar to cottage cheese.

Salsa:
A combination of tomato, chiles, and onions. Depending upon the chiles used, flavor ranges from mild to fiery hot.

Sapodilla:
A fruit with a rough, brown skin and sweet slightly grainy flesh. Eaten when fully ripe.

Sapota:
Also called the Mexican custard apple, sapotas resemble green apples in appearance. Clusters of the fruit are large and greenish-yellow.

Sofrito:
A combination of onions, garlic, cilantro, sweet chiles, and annato seeds. It serves as a base for many dishes as well as an all-purpose sauce.

Sopa:
Side dish consisting of rice, pasta, and sometimes tomatoes cooked in consommé. It can also be a dessert when sweet Spanish bread is added.

Spanish rice:
White rice sautéed in a skillet with tomatoes, green peppers, onions, and seasonings.

Spanish sauce:
Diced peppers, either mild or hot, are soaked, seeded, and ground to a paste. Herbs, spices, vegetables, and meat or poultry stock are added to make a fairly heavy paste or puree.

Taco:
A crisp, deep-fried corn tortilla folded in half to hold seasoned ground beef, diced tomatoes, shredded lettuce, and cheese.

Tamales:
Extruded, cooked corn flour wrapped around a chili beef filling. A sauce of chili con carne, tomato, or cheese can be used as an accompaniment.

Tomatillos:
Commonly known as ground tomatoes, they are small, firm, round, husk-covered green vegetables.

Tortilla:
The bread of Mexico. Baked, flat, round, thin cakes of unleavened cornmeal (masa) or wheat flour.

Tostadas:
Tortillas that have been fried until golden brown and crisp in hot lard or oil. They are served with various combinations of meat, poultry, sauces, chiles, lettuce, and tomatoes.

Verdolaga (purslane):
Vegetable with tender leaves and young stalks that can be eaten in a salad or cooked like spinach.

Yautia:
A starchy, edible tuber that is cooked and eaten like yams or potatoes.

CHAPTER 21

Exchanges Italiano

For some of our favorite foods, such as pizza and spaghetti, Americans are beholden to Italy. One of the most enjoyable aspects of Italian cooking is its diversity, which reflects the country's varied geography and climate. From Genoa in the north to Sicily in the south, Italy's regions use their native ingredients to create a dizzying and delicious array of dishes.

Northern Italy is the principal producer of meat, butter, and cheese, and these foods are a major part of the northern diet. Rice dishes such as risotto are also widely eaten, as is polenta, a cornmeal porridge. Pasta, such as ravioli, is usually stuffed with cheese or bits of meat and topped with a cream sauce. The area around Genoa is best known for pesto sauce, which is a basil, cheese, and nut paste usually served with pasta. Lighter foods, such as fresh vegetables prepared with herbs and olive oil, are also common.

Just to the south, in Tuscany, fish and vegetables are simply prepared using wine, olive oil, and fresh herbs. Florence is famous for its green spinach noodles, which are served with butter and grated Parmesan cheese. The term *Florentine* refers to a dish garnished with or containing finely chopped spinach. Rome is probably best known for fettuccine Alfredo, long egg noodles mixed with butter, cream, and grated cheese.

The southernmost regions of Italy, including the Mediterranean coast and the island of Sicily, are known for their diet of low-fat, low-cholesterol foods. Pasta, grains, vegetables, dried beans, and fish—prepared with little oil—are the cuisine of southern Italy. Pasta is usually unfilled and served with a tomato sauce. Pizza is native to Naples. Another form of pizza is calzone, which is pizza dough folded over a filling of cheese, ham, and/or salami, then baked or fried.

Authentic Italian meals begin with the *antipasto*, which means "before the food." This is followed by the *primi* or first course, which is usually pasta but may be soup or rice. Next is the second course or *secondi*, which is fish, chicken, veal, or other meat. This

201

Good Choices

Bruschetta

Chicken cacciatore

Chicken in wine sauce

Chicken marsala

Chicken ravioli in marinara sauce

Cioppino

Foccacia

Green salad

Grilled meats

Italian bread

Italian ice

Linguine with white or red clam sauce

Marinated artichokes

Marinated calamari

Marsala sauce

Minestrone

Mussels marinara

Pasta in wine sauce

Pasta primavera

Pasta with marinara sauce (or other tomato-based sauce)

Polenta (without butter or cheese)

Risotto (without butter)

Roasted pepper salad

Steamed clams

Veal cacciatore

Zita bolognese

Zuppa de pesce

Go Easy

Alfredo sauce

Butter sauce

Cannelloni

Cannoli

Carbonara sauce

Cream sauces

Eggplant or chicken parmigiana

Fettuccine alfredo

Fried calamari

Lasagna

Prosciutto

Salami

Shrimp scampi

course is usually served with a vegetable. A salad, or *insalata*, follows the meal. In most American Italian restaurants, however, you're likely be served salad first and pasta for a main course.

Eating healthful Italian food means avoiding cream and cheese sauces and going easy on cheese and meat-stuffed pastas. Better choices are plain pastas, chicken, or fish topped with tomato sauce (such as marinara), vegetable sauce (such as primavera), white wine sauce, or lemon butter sauce (piccata). Parmesan cheese is relatively low-fat and is tasty sprinkled over pasta or chicken with tomato or marinara sauce. Although olive oil is popular—and, as fats go, healthy—remember that it contains 120 calories per tablespoon. Limit the amount you use.

Sample Italian Meal

Menu	Exchanges
Minestrone soup, 1 cup	1 starch, 1 fat
Italian bread with garlic butter, 1 slice	1 starch, 1 fat
Veal cacciatore, 1 cutlet with sauce served on spaghetti	3 starch, 3 lean meat, 1 fat
Insalata di casa with low-calorie Italian dressing, 1 side salad	1 veg, 0–1 fat
Italian ice, ½ cup	1½ other carb

Meal Total

Exchanges:	5 starch, 1 veg, 1½ other carb, 3 lean meat, 3–4 fat
Calories:	850
Carbohydrate:	100 grams (46%)
Protein:	40 grams (21%)
Fat:	30 grams (33%)

ITALIAN FOOD LIST

Food	Quantity	Carbohydrate Choices	Exchanges
Starch			
Alfredo sauce	½ cup	1½	1½ starch, 1 med. fat meat, 2 fat
Bolognese sauce	½ cup	1	1 starch, 1 fat
Gazpacho	1½ cup	1	1 starch
Gnocchi	2 small	1	1 starch
Italian bread	1 slice (1 oz)	1	1 starch
Italian bread with garlic butter	1 slice (1 oz)	1	1 starch, 1–2 fat
Marinara sauce	½ cup	1	1 starch, 1 fat
Meat-flavored or mushroom spaghetti sauce	½ cup	1	1 starch, 1 fat
Minestrone soup	1 cup	1	1 starch, 1 fat
Pasta	½ cup	1	1 starch
Red clam sauce	1 cup	1	1 starch, 1 fat
Spaghetti sauce	½ cup	1	1 starch
Spaghetti sauce with meat	½ cup	1	1 starch, 1 med. fat meat
Vermicelli soup	1 cup	1	1 starch
Other Carbohydrates			
Italian ice	½ cup	1½	1½ other carb
Spumoni	½ cup	1	1 other carb, 2 fat
Vegetable			
Gazpacho	½ cup	0	1 veg
Italian green beans	½ cup	0	1 veg
Pizza sauce	¼ cup	0	1 veg
Ratatouille	½ cup	0	1 veg, 1 fat
Tomato paste	2 Tbsp	0	1 veg
Tomato puree	¼ cup	0	1 veg
Tomato sauce	⅓ cup	0	1 veg
Meat			
Italian sausage	1 oz	0	1 high fat meat
Meatballs	1 meatball (2" across)	0	1 med. fat meat

Food	Quantity	Carbohydrate Choices	Exchanges
Prosciutto (Italian ham)	1 oz	0	1 med. fat meat
Veal cutlet	1 oz	0	1 lean meat
White clam sauce	½ cup	0	1 high fat meat

Fat

Food	Quantity	Carbohydrate Choices	Exchanges
Alfredo sauce	2 Tbsp (1 oz)	0	2 fat
Italian dressing	1 Tbsp	0	1 fat
Olive oil	1 Tbsp	0	2 fat
Pesto sauce	2 Tbsp (1 oz)	0	3 fat

Combination Foods

Food	Quantity	Carbohydrate Choices	Exchanges
Antipasto	1 serving	0	2 veg, 2 high fat meat, 1 fat
Cannelloni	4 medium	2	2 starch, 3 med. fat meat, 2–3 fat
Cannelloni Florentine (with veal and spinach)	4 medium	2	2 starch, 2 med. fat meat, 2 fat
Chicken cacciatore	½ small breast	1	1 starch, 3 lean meat, 1 fat
Chicken parmigiana with noodles	½ small breast + 1 cup noodles	1	1 starch, 1 veg, 3 lean meat, 1 fat
Chicken or turkey tetrazzini (pollo alla tetrazzini)	1 cup	2	2 starch, 1 veg, 2 med. fat meat
Eggplant parmigiana	1 cup	1	1 starch, 1 veg, 2 med. fat meat, 1 fat
Fettuccine alfredo	1½ cup	2	2 starch, 6 fat
Fettuccine primavera	1½ cup	2	2 starch, 1 veg, 1 med. fat meat, 2 fat
Fettuccine with chicken	1 cup	2	2 starch, 2 med. fat meat, 1 fat
Lasagna			
Cheese or beef	3 x 4" piece	1	1 starch, 1 veg, 2 med. fat meat
Sausage	3 x 4" piece	2	2 starch, 3 med. fat meat, 3 fat

Food	Quantity	Carbohydrate Choices	Exchanges
Linguini with white clam sauce	1 cup	3	3 starch, 1 med. fat meat, 2–3 fat
Manicotti			
With ricotta and tomato sauce	2 shells	3	3 starch, 2 med. fat meat, 2 fat
With ricotta and meat	2 shells	3	3 starch, 3 med. fat meat, 2 fat
Pasta			
With marinara sauce	1 cup	3	3 starch, 1 fat
With meat sauce	1 cup	2	2 starch, 1 veg, 1 med. fat meat, 1 fat
Pizza			
Meat	1/8 of a 16–18 oz pizza	1	1 starch, 1 veg, 1 med. fat meat, 2 fat
Vegetarian	1/8 of a 16–18 oz pizza	2	2 starch, 1 veg, 2 fat
Ravioli			
Beef	1 cup	2	2 starch, 1 veg, 1 med. fat meat
Cheese	1 cup	2	2 starch, 1 veg, 1 med. fat meat, 2 fat
Shrimp primavera	1½ cup	0	2 veg, 3–4 lean meat, 2 fat
Spaghetti			
With meatballs	½ cup pasta with 6 small meatballs	2	2 starch, 1 veg, 2 med. fat meat
With tomato sauce	1 cup	3	3 starch, 1 veg
Tortellini	1 cup	2	2 starch, 2 veg, 2 fat
Veal cacciatore	1 cutlet with 1 cup spaghetti and ½ cup marinara sauce	3	3 starch, 3 lean meat, 1 fat
Veal marsala	1 cutlet	0	1 veg, 3 lean meat
Veal parmigiana	1 cutlet	2	2 starch, 1 veg, 3 lean meat, 1 fat

WORD LIST

Alfredo:
: A creamy cheese sauce.

Antipasto:
: Spicy Italian meats, seafoods, and/or vegetables arranged on a platter and served cold as an appetizer.

Arborio rice:
: An Italian short-grain rice that when cooked has the ability to absorb large amounts of liquid and still retain a firm texture.

Balsamic vinegar:
: Vinegar made from the juice of white grapes. Its dark color and sweet/sour flavor come from aging for several years in wooden barrels.

Bolognese:
: Named after the town of Bologna, Italy, it refers to dishes served with a thick, full-bodied meat and tomato-based sauce. Wine or cream are sometimes added.

Bruschetta:
: Pizza or bread dough seasoned with herbs and baked. Served in wedges with toppings such as chopped tomatoes and garlic.

Cannelloni:
: Hollow pasta filled with ricotta cheese, meat, and/or spinach and served with cheese and tomato sauce.

Caper:
: The unopened flower bud on a bush native to the Mediterranean region. Gathered and sun-dried, they are preserved by pickling in a vinegar brine or packed in salt, which gives them a pungent flavor.

Carbonara:
: A bacon, egg, and cheese sauce served with pasta.

Chicken cacciatore:
: Sautéed chicken pieces simmered in a meatless tomato sauce.

Cioppino:
: An elaborate fish stew.

Fettuccine Alfredo:
: Thin, flat pasta served with a creamy cheese sauce.

Florentine:
: A dish garnished with or containing finely ground spinach.

Foccacia:
: A flat, round bread sometimes flavored with herbs.

Frittatta:
: Italian omelet topped with sautéed vegetables and/or sausage.

Fusilli primavera:
: Spiral, long pasta topped with sautéed vegetables.

Gazpacho:
: A pureed vegetable soup usually served cold.

Gnocchi:
: Little dumplings made from white flour, potato, or a combination of both, and often topped with sauce.

Italian green beans:
: Wide, quick-cooking green beans often served in a sauce.

Kalamato olives:
: Black Greek olives slit so the wine-vinegar mixture in which they are soaked will penetrate.

Lasagna:
: Very wide, flat pasta layered with meat, cheese, and tomato sauce.

Manicotti:
: Large, tubular pasta filled with meat or cheese and served with meatless tomato sauce.

Marinara sauce:	A meatless Italian tomato sauce made with garlic, onions, and oregano.
Marsala:	A sweet dessert wine often used in preparations or desserts.
Minestrone:	A thick vegetable and pasta soup.
Parmigiana:	A granular textured parmesan cheese that is aged two years.
Pasta:	Fresh or dried flour-based noodles available in a variety of shapes, including fettuccine, linguine, spaghetti, cannelloni, macaroni, elbow, shells, rigatoni, rotelle, vermicelli, etc.
Pesce:	Seafood.
Pesto:	A basil, cheese, and nut paste usually served with pasta.
Polenta:	Cornmeal and water mixture, baked and served with a sauce.
Primavera:	Sautéed vegetables.
Prosciutto:	An Italian ham that has been salt-cured, seasoned and air-dried (not smoked). It is pressed to produce a firm texture and is sliced very thin.
Ratatouille:	Tomatoes, eggplant, and zucchini cooked in olive oil.
Ravioli:	A pasta square stuffed with eggs, vegetables, cheese, or meat and covered with tomato sauce.
Risotto:	Italian short-grain rice that has a creamy consistency when cooked; often mixed with butter and cheese before serving.
Shrimp scampi:	Large shrimp seasoned with oil.
Spumoni:	Chocolate and vanilla ice cream with a layer of rum-flavored whipped cream containing nuts and fruit.
Veal cacciatore:	Veal cutlet topped with tomato sauce and sautéed onions, mushrooms and peppers.
Veal parmigiana:	Thin slices of veal, pounded for tenderness, rolled in bread crumbs and Parmesan cheese, and covered with mozzarella cheese and a meatless tomato sauce.
Veal piccata:	Medallions of veal lightly sautéed in a butter, lemon, and wine sauce.
White clam sauce:	White-wine-based cream sauce containing whole clams.
Zuppe:	Soup.
Zuppa de pesce:	Fish soup.

CHAPTER 22

Spicy Indian Exchanges

When many of us think of Indian food, we think "hot and spicy." But as in other cuisines, there is remarkable diversity within Indian cooking, and the level of heat differs from region to region. Foods from south India use a lot of chiles, can be very hot, and are likely to include fish and rice. Foods from north India are tamer, relying primarily on breads and dahls (sauces made from pureed beans or lentils). Vegetarianism is common throughout all of India, ranging from the simple exclusion of beef to the elimination of all meat, poultry, fish, and eggs.

The raw ingredients of Indian food vary widely. A range of whole and split lentils, dried beans, and dried peas are included and are a significant source of protein and calories. Vegetables such as onions, peppers, potatoes, and tomatoes are also common, as are chicken and seafood. Basmati rice, a fragrant, long-grain, premium white rice unique to Indian cooking accompanies most meals, as do breads. Coconuts, common in some parts of India, also make a frequent appearance as coconut milk, coconut cream, and shredded coconut. Milk and dairy products such as buttermilk, curds, and cottage cheese are used as bases for curries, snack foods and desserts. Plain, low-fat yogurt is frequently used in gravies and sauces.

The food preparation style we most often associate with India is "curry," but the single spice that Americans call curry is unknown in Indian cooking. In India, curry is a blend of fragrant ground spices, and there are many different recipes for curry. Families guard and hand down curry recipes for generations. Garam masala is one type of curry, containing cardamom, coriander, cumin, cloves, cinnamon, and black pepper. "Curry" also refers to a dish made with one of these spice blends. A curry dish may consist of meat, poultry, fish, potatoes, vegetables, dahl, or combinations of these. Other spices commonly used in Indian cooking are mint, garlic, and ginger. In southern Indian dishes, chiles and pepper are also added to dishes to give them a hot taste.

Ovens and baking are rarely used in Indian cooking. If an oven is used, it is often a clay oven called a tandoor, which cooks with charcoal. More often, an Indian dish will start with vegetables sautéed in oil. Then, meat or poultry is added along with ingredients such as yogurt or coconut milk, and the mixture is cooked to integrate all the flavors. Other common cooking methods are stewing, frying, boiling, and steaming. Main dishes such as masala, curries, and bhunas are stewed. Appetizers and breads are often fried, although some breads are cooked on a griddle without fat.

In some homes, foods may be served family style. Breads and small bowls of the curry dishes are placed on a thali (a large metal platter) in the middle of the table. Several bowls of condiments— for example, hot onion relish, chutney, dahl, tamarind sauce, and raita—are usually included as well. Everyone takes a portion from the thali, but each person has a separate, large bowl of rice. Desserts are generally not an important part of Indian cuisine. A dinner might end with chai, a beverage usually prepared with black tea, milk, and cardamom. Darjeeling tea is a variety of tea native to India.

In Indian restaurants, soup and appetizers are usually served first. Next, the breads, rice, and entrée selections are served. Vegetables and legumes, including lentils and chickpeas, play an important role in entrées. Common vegetables include spinach, eggplant, cabbage, potatoes, and peas; onions, green peppers, and tomatoes are often found in stewed entrées. Vegetables are incorporated into many dishes, including curries, biryani, and pullas.

The first challenge of enjoying Indian food in restaurants is learning the names used in Indian cuisine. Often you may find menu listings spelled differently by several letters. For example, you may see vandaloo or vindaloo, samosa or samoosa, raita or rayte, dahl or dal. The second challenge is keeping fat intake under control, as fat is frequently used in food preparation. Ghee (clarified butter) is a common ingredient for frying and sautéing; this is the only animal fat used in Indian cooking. Vegetable oils—usually sesame, peanut, or coconut oil—are also used in sautéing. Most appetizers are fried, and the initial step in preparing many entrée dishes is sautéing onions and other ingredients in oil or ghee. Still, there are many healthy Indian foods—you just need to learn how to spot them.

Good Choices

Baked breads such as chappati, naan, or phulka

Brown or basmati rice

Curried chicken or fish

Curried lentils and chickpeas

Dahl

Fruit and vegetable chutneys

Raita

Tandoori chicken or fish

Yogurt-based sauces and curries

Go Easy

Chicken or cheese pakoras

Dishes using cream, coconut oil, or milk

Fried breads such as puri, paratha, or puppodum

Korma dishes

Koulfi

Samosas

Sample Indian Meal

Menu	Exchanges
Puppodum, 2 small	1 starch
Tandoori murgh (barbecued chicken), 4 oz	4 lean meat, 1 fat
Alu matar (potato and pea curry), ½ cup	1 starch, 1 fat
Piaz aur tamatar ka salad (onions and tomato salad), 1 medium	1 veg
Naan, 1 small loaf	1½ starch
Basmati chawal rice, ½ cup	1 starch

Meal Total

Exchanges:	4½ starch, 1 veg, 4 lean meat, 2 fat
Calories:	700
Carbohydrate:	75 grams (41%)
Protein:	45 grams (25%)
Fat:	25 grams (34%)

INDIAN FOOD LIST

Food	Quantity	Carbohydrate Choices	Exchanges
Starch			
Alu mattar	1 cup	2	2 starch, 3 fat
Alu paratha	1 (6" across)	2½	2½ starch, 6 fat
Arhar, cooked	1 bowl (3" across)	1	1 starch
Arrowroot flour	2 Tbsp	1	1 starch
Barley, cooked	⅓ cup	1	1 starch
Basmati rice, cooked	½ cup	1	1 starch
Beet root	3 oz	1	1 starch
Chapati, 5–6" across	1 chapati	1	1 starch
Colocasia, cooked	¼ cup	1	1 starch
Dahl			
Uncooked	2 Tbsp	1	1 starch
Cooked	1 bowl (3" across)	1	1 starch
Dosa	1 (6" across)	1	1 starch
Idli	1 (3"across)	1	1 starch
Lentil soup	1 cup	1½	1½ starch, 1 fat
Lobia	1 small bowl	1	1 starch
Moong dal, cooked	1 medium bowl	1	1 starch
Naan	¼ large or 1 small loaf	1	1 starch
Noodles, cooked	½ cup	1	1 starch
Peas pullao	1 cup	3	3 starch
Phoa, uncooked	3 Tbsp	1	1 starch
Phulka	1 (6" across)	1	1 starch
Porridge	¾ cup	1	1 starch
Potato	½ medium	1	1 starch
Puppodum, plain	2 small	1	1 starch
Puri	1 (5" across)	1	1 starch, 2½ fat
Rajmah	½ cup	1	1 starch
Rice, cooked	⅓ cup	1	1 starch
Rice flour, uncooked	2 Tbsp	1	1 starch
Samosa, with potato filling	1 piece	1	1 starch, 2 fat
Saag paneer	1 cup	1	1 starch, 1 fat

Food	Quantity	Carbohydrate Choices	Exchanges
Upma, plain without vegetables, cooked	½ cup	1	1 starch
Whole wheat flour	3 Tbsp	1	1 starch
Fruit			
Ber (small apples)	5–8 fruits	1	1 fruit
Guava	1 medium or ½ cup	1	1 fruit
Loquat	5–6 fruits	1	1 fruit
Mango	½ medium	1	1 fruit
Papaya	½ fruit	1	1 fruit
Milk			
Carol	1 cup	1	1 milk, 1 ½ fat
Dahi (curds)	1 cup	1	1 milk
Khoa	2 Tbsp	1	1 milk, 1 ½ fat
Vegetable			
Ashgourd, cooked	½ cup	0	1 veg
Bottle gourd, cooked	1 ⅓ cup	0	1 veg
Bhindi	½ cup	0	1 veg
Brinjal	¾ cup	0	1 veg
Capsicum	¾ cup	0	1 veg
Chow chow, cooked	½ cup	0	1 veg
Drumstick, cooked	½ cup	0	1 veg
Lady fingers (okra)	½ cup	0	1 veg
Lauki	¾ cup	0	1 veg
Onion chutney	¼ cup	0	1 veg
Raita	½ cup	0	1 veg
Tamata salet	½ cup	0	1 veg
Tori	¾ cup	0	1 veg
Meat/Meat Substitutes			
Chana dahl	½ cup	0	2 lean meat, 2 fat
Chicken tandoori	4 oz	0	4 lean meat, 1 fat
Lamb, chicken, fish, mutton, pork	1 oz	0	1 med. fat meat
Pakora, potato and chickpea flour	2 balls (1" across)	0	1 high fat meat, 3 fat

Food	Quantity	Carbohydrate Choices	Exchanges
Paneer			
Made with skim milk	¼ cup	0	1 lean meat
Made with whole milk	¼ cup	0	1 high fat meat
Fat			
Coconut, grated, unsweetened	2 Tbsp	0	1 fat
Coconut chutney	2 Tbsp	0	1 fat
Coconut oil	1 tsp	0	1 fat
Ghee	1 tsp	0	1 fat
Oil (maize, refined, saffola, or soya)	1 tsp	0	1 fat
Combination Foods			
Biryani	1½ cups	3	3 starch, 1 veg, 2 lean meat, 1 fat
Kheema do pyaza med. fat meat, 2 fat	1 cup	1	1 starch, 3
Kofta	3 balls (1½" across)	0	3 med. fat meat, 5 fat
Machli aur tamatar	3 oz	1	1 starch, 3 med. fat meat, 1 fat
Masala dosa	1 large	2	2 starch, 4 fat
Mattar paneer	½ cup	1	1 starch, 1 high fat meat, 3 fat
Murgh kari (chicken curry)	3 oz chicken	1	1 starch, 3 med. fat meat
Samosa			
Filled with lamb	1 medium (2½")	1	1 starch, 1 med. fat meat, 2 fat
Filled with peas and potatoes	1 medium (2½")	2	2 starch, 2 fat

WORD LIST

Achar:	Brine-pickled fruits and vegetables, e.g., limes, lemons, mangoes, green beans, and green chiles.
Alu mattar:	Curried potatoes and peas.
Alu paratha:	Flat whole wheat bread with spiced potato filling.
Appam:	Deep fried pancake made of rice, lentils, and flour.
Ashgourd:	Pumpkinlike vegetable with light green skin and white flesh.
Asafetida:	A strong-smelling sap or resin from the roots of various East Indian plants. Powdered, it is used in very small amounts in lentil dishes and meat stews.
Balushahi:	Crisp, sweet pastry fried in ghee, then dipped in sugar syrup.
Barfi:	Sweet with a fudgelike texture made from milk and sugar and flavored with vanilla or cardamom.
Besan:	Chickpea flour.
Bhindi:	Okra.
Bhuna:	Chicken, beef, or lamb roasted with spices, onions, and tomatoes.
Biryani:	Shrimp, lamb, or vegetable layered with basmati rice and vegetables.
Bottle gourd:	Pale green, large bulb-shaped, thick skinned vegetable with thick pulp.
Cardamom:	Spice made from the dried fruit of a plant of the ginger family. The pods or seeds are used in meat, rice, and some dessert dishes. One of the most expensive but common spices used in curries.
Chana dahl:	Dahl made from chickpeas.
Chapati:	Thin, grilled, whole-wheat bread made without fat.
Chicken tikka:	Bite-size pieces of chicken cooked in clay ovens with charcoal.
Chole:	Chickpeas. Aloo chole is chickpeas cooked with tomatoes and potatoes.
Chow chow:	Small bulblike vegetable with rough, light-green skin and white pulp.
Chutney:	Highly seasoned relish or accompaniment made from raw, cooked, or pickled fruits or vegetables and/or coconut.
Coconut milk:	A creamy liquid extracted by grating fresh coconut meat (not the liquid inside the coconut).
Colocasia:	Lotuslike plant that grows in water or marshy places. Cooked and used as a vegetable.
Curry:	A mixture of individually roasted spices.
Dahi (curds):	Unflavored yogurt eaten at most Indian meals as an accompaniment, either plain or mixed with vegetables.

Dahl (dal), raw:	Raw dahl is a pulse (edible seed) resembling the common split pea. Dahl also refers to a light, spicy puree made of many kinds of dried beans, peas or lentils; for example, chana dahl is made from chickpeas; mung dahl is made from mung beans.
Dosa:	Pancake-like bread made from fermented rice flour and lentils and sometimes stuffed with vegetables.
Drumstick:	Narrow, long, fibrous green vegetable used in curries.
Fennel:	Another spice used in curries, also referred to as sweet cumin. Commonly used in sweet dishes or tea.
Firni:	A sweet pudding made of milk, cream of rice, and nuts.
Garam masala:	A blend of dried ground spices, usually black peppers, cumin, coriander, cloves, ginger, cinnamon and others.
Ghee:	Butter that has been clarified or gently warmed over low heat until it browns lightly, giving it a distinct aroma. It is used as a flavoring or as a topping for rice and breads.
Halva:	A very sweet dessert made from milk, vegetables such as carrots or pumpkin, and sometimes nuts.
Idli:	A flattened, cupcake-shaped bread made from ground lentils and rice, and steamed in small saucers.
Kheema mattar:	Curried ground lamb or beef and peas cooked in a spicy sauce.
Kheema do pyaza:	Curried ground lamb or beef with onions.
Khir (kheer):	Sweet pudding made of milk and long-grain rice and flavored with cardamom.
Kofta:	Vegetables, cheese, and ground meat such as lamb that is shaped like a meatball, fried and curried.
Korma:	A curried dish with a thickened nut-and-yogurt sauce.
Kulcha:	Leavened baked bread.
Lauki:	A bottle gourd.
Lobia:	Black-eyed peas.
Loquat:	A small, round fruit with yellow-orange skin and pale yellow to orange flesh with black seeds. The flavor is like a blend of banana and pineapple.
Machli aur tamatar:	Curried halibut.
Malai:	A thick cream that is made from milk by separating and collecting the top part of boiled milk. Used in entrées for a thick, creamy sauce.
Masala:	Chicken, beef, lamb, fish, or shrimp cooked in a thick spicy yogurt and curry sauce.
Masala dosa:	A crepelike pancake with spiced potato filling.
Mattar paneer:	Green peas with cottage cheese.
Naan (nan):	Individual leavened flat bread made of white flour, and traditionally baked in a clay oven.

Pakora:	Deep fried, spicy vegetables (cauliflower, eggplant, potato, lentils, etc.) or chicken fritters.
Paneer:	Homemade cottage cheese used in curries, vegetable and rice dishes, and desserts. Made from milk that is curdled with lemon juice and then strained through cheese cloth.
Paratha:	Unleavened bread made from wheat flour and cooked on a grill. It may be spread with oil or butter during or after cooking. Parathas can also be stuffed with vegetables such as potatoes, cauliflower, radish, spinach, or dahl.
Phoa:	Rice that has been pounded into ragged, translucent flakes. Eaten with milk as a cold cereal, or plain or deep-fried as a snack.
Phulka:	Puffed, whole-wheat, round bread, made without fat and cooked directly over a very low gas flame.
Pulse:	The edible seeds of various leguminous crops such as peas, beans, or lentils.
Puppodums (papadam):	Very light, puffed, crisp wafers made from spicy lentils and served as a side dish or appetizer.
Pullaos:	Plain pullao is basmati rice cooked with saffron; peas pullao is basmati rice cooked with peas and spices; shrimp pullao is basmati rice cooked with shrimp and spices.
Puri:	Thin, deep-fried, whole-wheat bread.
Rajmah:	Curried, cooked red beans.
Raita:	Saladlike combination of yogurt with grated cucumbers (or other raw or cooked vegetables), onions, and spices.
Ras malai:	Paneer (cheese) balls boiled in condensed milk and sugar.
Roti:	Indian breads, including chapati, dosa, idli, kulcha, naan, paratha, phulka, and puri (see individual definitions).
Saag paneer:	Spinach cooked with cottage cheese.
Saffron:	Spice obtained by drying the threadlike, deep-orange stamens of the saffron crocus. Known as the most expensive spice in the world, saffron is used in small quantities in Indian cooking.
Sambhar:	Lentil puree cooked with vegetables and spices.
Samosa:	Deep-fried pastry filled with a mixture of vegetables or meat.
Shami kebab:	Fried patty made of ground meat.
Shrikhand:	A sweet made of curds, sugar, and flavoring such as cardamom.
Tamarind:	Fruit with a long, flattened, cinnamon-brown pod. Usually used dried or as pulp in cooking to impart a sweet-sour taste.

Tamata salat:	Diced tomatoes and onions with hot spices and lemon.
Tandoori:	Cylindrical clay ovens heated with charcoal.
Tandoori chicken:	Chicken roasted in clay ovens with charcoal. Tandoori chicken has a red color on top from the spices and cooking.
Turmeric:	A spice from the ginger family that gives the yellow-orange color to commercial curry.
Upma:	A breakfast item made with cream of wheat or fuji spices, and sometimes with vegetables.
Vindaloo:	Chicken, beef, lamb, or fish cooked with potatoes and hot spices.

CHAPTER 23

Exchanges for
Jewish Cookery

The eating traditions of Jewish people are based on the laws of
Kashrut, which are the general dietary laws from the Torah. The
Torah is the Jewish book of laws and their interpretations, encom-
passing the five books of Moses and the customs for celebrating Jewish holidays. These laws of Kashrut are observed in varying degrees
by orthodox, conservative, and reformed denominations.

"Kosher," defined as "proper," or "fit," or "in accordance with
religious law," is used to describe the specific dietary and lifestyle
guidelines sanctioned by Jewish law. For example, kosher laws
dictate how animals are slaughtered and how meat is prepared, as
well as the way various meals are prepared and served. The word
"traif," which describes animals found non-kosher because of
physical damage or imperfections, is commonly used to describe
all foods that are non-kosher, not just meats.

A crucial aspect of planning meals according to the laws of
Kashrut is the separation of meat (fleischig) or poultry from dairy
foods (milchig). Dairy and meat or poultry products may not be
eaten at the same meal. After eating meat, kosher households must
wait one to six hours before eating any dairy products. Dairy products may be eaten first; however, the diner must rinse out his or her
mouth and wait one-half to one hour before eating meat. In kosher
households, not only are meat and dairy foods separated; the dishes and utensils used for meat and dairy meals are also separated.
This is known as "keeping kosher."

Meats that are acceptable come from animals that chew their
cud, have split hooves (cattle, sheep, goats, and deer), have been
slaughtered in a kosher manner, and have had the additional step
of being koshered through a soaking and salting process. Chicken,
turkey, goose, pheasant, and duck are kosher, and only eggs from
kosher birds are allowed. Fish that have both fins and scales are

considered kosher and do not require a ritual slaughtering and additional koshering. Pig and pork products are not kosher, nor are birds of prey.

"Pareve" foods, or neutral foods, are foods that contain neither meat nor dairy products. These foods may be served at either meat or dairy meals and are prepared in utensils used for pareve only. All fruits, vegetables, starches, and eggs are pareve, as are many breads, cakes, and cereals. Fish are also considered pareve.

Many food companies prepare food products that are kosher certified, so kosher convenience foods are widely available. On Kosher food labels you'll find a "U," which represents the Union of Orthodox Jewish Congregations of America (UOJCA). This is a national kosher certification program operated in conjunction with the Rabbinical Council of America, which certifies more than 15,000 products. The letter "K" may also be used to denote kosher foods.

Historically, the kosher diet has been high in fat. Many cuts of kosher meat are well-marbled with fat. Schmaltz (chicken fat) is used for flavor and sometimes as an ingredient in sandwiches. Fried dishes like blintzes (crepes) and matzo brie (fried matzo) also are popular in kosher cooking. In place of schmaltz or butter, you

Good Choices	**Go Easy**
Bagels	Bubke
Bean soup	Hamantaschen (purim tart)
Borscht	Hot dogs
Cabbage soup	Knockwurst
Chicken noodle or chicken rice soup	Kuchen and Mandel Bread
Gefilte fish plate	Lekach
Lox	Pastrami
Rye and pumpernickel breads	Rugalah
Split pea soup	Schmaltz
Stewed fruits	Teiglach
Turkey breast or roast beef sandwiches	
Whole grains such as oatmeal, barley, brown rice, kasha	

can use small amounts of margarine or kosher certified vegetable oil, which are pareve (neutral). Many kosher meats and poultry tend to be high in sodium, because salting is part of the koshering process. Fresh kosher fish does not have to be salted to be kosher. In preparing your own dishes, you can use substitutes for high saturated fat and high salt products.

Sample Jewish Meal

Menu	Exchanges
Challah, 1 slice	1 starch
Gefilte fish, 2 oz	1 lean meat
Horseradish	free
Beet borscht, 1 cup	2 veg
Stewed chicken, 3 oz	3 high fat meat
Potato kugel, 1 cup	2 starch
Fruit compote, ½ cup	1 fruit

Meal Total

Exchanges:	3 starch, 1 fruit, 2 veg, 1 lean meat, 3 high fat meat
Calories:	700
Carbohydrate:	70 grams (40%)
Protein:	40 grams (23%)
Fat:	30 grams (38%)

JEWISH FOOD LIST

Food	Quantity	Carbohydrate Choices	Exchanges
Starch			
Bagel	½ medium (1 oz)	1	1 starch
Bialy	½ medium (1 oz)	1	1 starch
Bulke	½ medium (1 oz)	1	1 starch
Challah (hallah)	1 slice (1 oz)	1	1 starch
Cream of Wheat®, cooked	½ cup	1	1 starch
Farfel, dry	3 Tbsp	1	1 starch
Hard roll	1 small	1	1 starch
Kasha (buckwheat groats)			
Cooked	¾ cup	2	2 starch
Dry	2 Tbsp	1	1 starch
Kichlach	3 (1" square)	1	1 starch
Lentils	⅓ cup	1	1 starch
Lokshen (noodles)	½ cup	1	1 starch
Matzo, thin (plain, honey spiced, unsalted, or whole wheat)	1 (1 oz)	1½	1½ starch
Matzo balls (knaidlach)	2 Tbsp dry or 2 prepared balls	1	1 starch
Matzo ball soup	1 cup	1	1 starch, 1 fat
Matzo chips or crisps	1 oz (½ cup)	1½	1½ starch
Matzo crackers, 1½" square	7 crackers (1 oz)	1	1 starch
Mini crackers	13 crackers (1 oz)	1½	1½ starch
Matzo farfel, dry	¼ cup	1	1 starch
Matzo kugel	½ serving	1	1 starch, 1 fat
Matzo meal	¼ cup	1½	1½ starch
Matzo meal pancakes	1 medium	1	1 starch, 2 fat
Noodle pudding	½ cup	1½	1½ starch
Potato knish	1 (3" across) or 2 small	1	1 starch, 2 fat
Potato kugel	½ cup	1	1 starch
Potato latkes (potato pancakes)	3 Tbsp batter or 3 prepared	1	1 starch
Potato starch (flour)	2 Tbsp	1	1 starch
Pumpernickel bread	1 slice	1	1 starch
Rye bread	1 slice	1	1 starch
Split peas, cooked	½ cup	1	1 starch

Food	Quantity	Carbohydrate Choices	Exchanges
Vegetable			
Borscht	½ cup	0	1 veg, 1 fat
Sauerkraut	½ cup	0	1 veg
Sorrel (schav)	½ cup	0	1 veg
Meat/Meat Substitutes			
Beef tongue	1 oz	0	1 med. fat meat
Brisket	1 oz	0	1 med. fat meat
Caviar	1 oz	0	1 lean meat
Chicken, stewed	1 oz	0	1 high fat meat
Corned beef	1 oz	0	1 med. fat meat
Flanken	1 oz	0	1 lean meat
Gefilte fish	2 oz	0	1 lean meat
Kippered herring	1 oz	0	1 lean meat
Livers, chopped	¼ cup	0	1 med. fat meat
Lox (smoked salmon)	1 oz	0	1 lean meat
Pastrami	1 oz	0	1 high fat meat
Pickled herring	1 oz	0	1 lean meat
Pot cheese	¼ cup	0	1 lean meat
Sablefish, smoked	1 oz	0	1 med. fat meat
Salmon, pink, canned in water	1 oz	0	1 very lean meat
Salmon, red, canned in water	1 oz	0	1 very lean meat
Sardines (canned, drained)	2 medium	0	1 lean meat
Fat			
Chicken fat (schmaltz)	1 tsp	0	1 fat
Cream cheese	1 Tbsp	0	1 fat
Grebenes	1 tsp	0	1 fat
Sour cream	2 Tbsp	0	1 fat
Light	3 Tbsp	0	1 fat
Free Foods			
Coffee whiteners			
Nondairy liquid	1 Tbsp	0	free
Nondairy powdered	2 tsp	0	free
Horseradish	–	0	free
Pickles, dill	1½ large	0	free

Food	Quantity	Carbohydrate Choices	Exchanges
Combination Foods			
Cabbage-beet borscht	1 cup	1	1 starch, 1 fat
Cheese blintzes, frozen	8 oz entrée	2	2 starch, 2 med. fat meat, 3 fat
Chicken and dumplings	1 cup	2	2 starch, 2 med. fat meat, 1 fat
Cholent with meat	1 cup	2	2 starch, 1 veg, 2 med. fat meat; 1–2 fat
Meatless	1 cup	3	3 starch, 1–2 veg, 1–2 fat
Kreplach, meat	2 small	1	1 starch, 2 med. fat meat
Lentil soup	1 cup	2	2 starch, 1 lean meat
Noodle pudding	½ cup	2	2 starch, 1 fat
Split pea soup	1 cup	2	2 starch, 1 lean meat
Stuffed cabbage in tomato sauce	1 large roll	1	1 starch, 1 veg, 2 med. fat meat
Tzimmes			
Carrot and apple	½ cup	2	2 starch
Sweet potato	½ cup	2	2 starch

WORD LIST

Bagel:	A hard yeast roll shaped like a doughnut.
Bialy:	A flat breakfast roll that is softer than a bagel.
Blintzes:	Very thin, rolled crepe usually filled with cottage cheese, pot cheese, or a fruit mixture.
Borscht:	Soup made with beets, cabbage, or other vegetables and sour cream. It may be served hot or cold.
Bubke:	Coffeecake that is yeast-risen and sweetened with cinnamon and sugar.
Bulke:	Large, light, yeast roll that is softer than a bagel.
Challah (hallah):	A loaf of very light egg bread, often braided and usually prepared for the Sabbath and holidays.
Cholent:	A slow-cooking stew that can be prepared with or without meat.
Farfel:	Noodle dough grated into barley-sized grains and served in soup.
Flanken:	Flank steak.
Fleischig:	Meat and meat products. Also used to describe meals that include meat.
Gefilte fish:	A highly seasoned chopped freshwater fish such as carp, pike, or whitefish mixture that is blended with eggs and matzo meal.
Grebenes:	Rendered chicken fat and chicken skin fried with onions.
Hamantaschen (purim tart):	Three-cornered cakes made with pastry or cookie crust and filled with poppy seeds, dried fruit, or cheese.
Kasha:	Buckwheat groats served as a cooked cereal or as a potato substitute.
Kashrut:	The Kosher dietary laws based on the Torah.
Kichlach:	Light egg cookies.
Kishke:	Beef casings stuffed with seasoned filling made from matzo, flour, fat, and onions.
Knaidlach:	Matzo balls made of matzo meal, eggs, and fat, usually served in chicken soup.
Knish:	Pastry (sometimes potato-based) filled with ground meat, potato, or kasha and spices.
Kreplach:	Bite-sized pastry filled with meat or cheese mixture, similar to ravioli.
Kuchen:	Coffeecake.
Kugel:	Pudding or casserole, commonly made with potatoes or noodles.
Latkes:	Pancakes. Potato latkes are very popular.
Leckach:	Honey cake.
Lokshen:	Noodles.
Lox:	Smoked, salted salmon that is cut very thin.

Matzo:	Flat, unleavened cracker.
Matzo farfel:	Barley-sized matzo grains.
Matzo meal:	Finely ground matzo used in cooking and baking.
Milchig:	Milk or dairy foods. Also used to describe meals that include dairy products.
Pareve:	Neutral foods such as fish, eggs, fruits, and vegetables, which may be served at either a meat or a dairy meal.
Pirogi or piroshkes:	Pastry filled with cheese or meat.
Pot cheese:	Cream cheese or other farmer-style cheese.
Rugalah (strudel):	Thin pastry rolled up in fruit and nut filling.
Sablefish:	Though it is commonly called "black cod," this northern Pacific fish is not cod. A high fat content gives it a soft texture and a rich taste that is surprisingly mild.
Schav:	Soup made from sorrel that is similar to borscht.
Schmaltz:	Rendered chicken fat, often used in cooking or pastry making.
Sorrel:	A member of the buckwheat family. Cooked as a green, leafy vegetable.
Teiglach:	Small balls of sweet dough cooked in honey.
Traif (trefe):	Foods that are non-kosher, forbidden, and ritually unfit.
Tzimmes:	Versatile, hot side dish often made with dried fruit, carrots, and sweet potatoes, and sweetened with honey. Tzimmes may be prepared with meat and served as a main dish or made with fruit and served as a dessert.

PART SIX

Exchanges on the Go

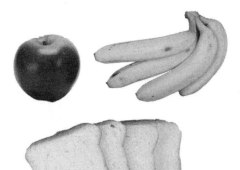

CHAPTER 24

Exchanges for the Fast Food Phenomenon

Accoring to a recent survey, more than half of us eat out or purchase food "to go" on an average day. Three out of every four away-from-home meals are eaten at fast-food restaurants, which is the most distinctively American part of the food service business. Can you choose fast foods that are not loaded with grease and calories? The answer, of course, is yes. With careful attention, you can eat healthfully *and* on-the-go.

The average calorie count of a fast-food meal is 685, which is not outrageously high. The key to making wise choices is to buy small- or regular-sized sandwiches, fries, and other items. Avoid the "jumbo," "giant," or "deluxe" versions—larger serving sizes mean not only additional calories but also more fat, cholesterol, and sodium. The chart below shows the maximum amount of calories, fat, and sodium you should consume in one fast food meal.

	Calories/Meal	Fat/Meal (grams)	Sodium/Meal (milligrams)
Women	500–600	20–25	1000
Men	800–900	30–35	1000

Some fast food restaurants provide nutrition information for their menu items, which makes sticking to these guidelines easier. Studies of fast food chains show remarkable uniformity in the portion sizes and nutritional value of menu items. This means that it may be easier to know what you're getting in a fast food meal than in some gourmet restaurant meals. Here are some suggestions to help you make smart choices.

Burgers: Bigger Isn't Better

To keep the fat and calorie content of burgers under control, scale down to single-patty selections. Choose a plain, regular hamburger, and skip the cheese, special sauces, and mayonnaise-based dressings. If you've got a double-decker appetite, pile on the lettuce and tomato for a satisfying and healthy sandwich. To accompany your burger, get a side salad or regular french fries (not super-sized!). Here's an example of the difference these choices can make:

Burger Meal 1	Burger Meal 2
Deluxe hamburger with special sauce, large fries, large chocolate chip cookie	Quarter pound hamburger, regular fries, diet soft drink
1200 calories	630 calories
64 grams of fat	43 grams of fat
1385 milligrams of sodium	770 milligrams of sodium

Chicken and Fish: Breading Traps the Fat

Battering, breading, or deep-frying chicken or fish cancels out their usual low-fat advantage. If fried chicken is your only choice, choose regular coating over extra crispy varieties (which soak up more oil during cooking). Even better, peel off the skin and lose 100 calories plus most of the fat and excess sodium. The example below shows the impact of different cooking methods on the final food.

Chicken Sandwich 1	Chicken Sandwich 2
Breaded, deep-fried chicken sandwich	Grilled chicken sandwich
500–700 calories	300–450 calories
30–40 grams of fat	7–25 grams of fat
1000 milligrams of sodium	900 milligrams of sodium

Likewise, baked fish has half the fat and calories of fried fish and is lower in sodium. Skip the tartar sauce and use cocktail sauce or lemon juice instead. Two tablespoons of tartar sauce provide 200 calories. An equal amount of cocktail sauce provides thirty-five calories, and lemon juice has no calories. Each adds a nice flavor to fish. For side dishes, order mashed potatoes with a small amount of gravy instead of french fries and you'll save 200 calories.

Pizza: Extra Toppings, Extra Calories

As a snack or quick meal, pizza can fit nicely into a well-balanced diet. It's not necessarily a low-calorie food, but its calories contribute very respectably to nutrition. Two slices of a thin-crust sixteen-inch cheese pizza contain 375 calories, and only twenty-four percent of the calories are from fat. By selecting thin-crust pizza instead of pan or thick-crust, you save up to 130 calories per slice. When choosing toppings, stay with mushrooms, onions, green or hot peppers, and other vegetable toppings. Extra cheese, pepperoni, and sausage mean extra fat and calories—as much as 170 calories per slice. To avoid extra sodium, skip the olives and anchovies.

Plain Baked Potato: A Great Choice

A plain baked potato is nourishing, filling, and virtually free of fat and sodium. A large plain potato provides 250 calories and two grams of fat. When topped with one-quarter cup cottage cheese or one to two tablespoons of grated Swiss, cheddar, or Parmesan cheese and paired with a salad, a baked potato becomes a complete meal. However, beware of other common potato toppings—cheese sauce, crumbled bacon, and sour cream can increase the fat level from two grams to as much as forty grams. Calories can increase from 250 to 590. A deluxe, super-stuffed baked potato with sour cream, butter, bacon, and cheese has 648 calories and six teaspoons of fat!

Salad: A Healthy Complement

A salad bar is a healthy alternative to high-fat fast food sandwiches, and many restaurants now offer a trip to the salad bar on their menus. As you fill your plate, go heavy on raw vegetables and pass on prepared salads such as potato salad, pasta salad, and taco salad. Some fast food restaurants also have pre-made salads on their menus. The best choice is a grilled chicken or a garden salad; avoid chef salads, which include meats, cheeses, and eggs that boost the fat content.

As with all fast foods, salads have their pitfalls—there's no quicker way to cancel out the health advantages of a salad than to drown it in regular salad dressing. Instead, stick with low-calorie, reduced-fat dressings. A large salad containing a variety of vegetables, one-half cup cottage cheese, and a light salad dressing has less than 250 calories; adding just one tablespoon of regular dressing, some bacon bits, and one-quarter cup macaroni or potato salad doubles the calories to 500.

Sandwiches: Many Low-Fat Options

Turkey, ham, and roast beef sandwiches are good fast food choices, as long as you stick to the regular and junior-sized versions instead of the deluxe versions. Lettuce, tomato, peppers, and other fresh vegetables add nutrients as well as a pleasing crunch to make a sandwich healthy and satisfying. It's best to avoid mayonnaise and mayonnaise-based toppings, which can 100 calories or more per tablespoon. Use mustard, horseradish, or barbecue sauce instead. Croissant sandwiches are deceptively high in fat, averaging 400 to 600 calories. Stick with a sandwich on regular or whole-grain bread, a bun, or pita bread and save from 150 to 300 calories.

Mexican Food: Surprisingly Healthy

Entrées made with soft flour tortillas are generally better choices than those made with fried (hard) corn tortillas, but a small taco or tostada accompanied by tomatoes and fresh vegetables can be a good choice. Chicken or vegetable burritos, in particular, are healthy, low-fat choices. To keep the fat down, skip the sour cream and guacamole and pile on extra salsa, tomatoes, and lettuce. Cheese and refried beans also can add a lot of fat, so they need to be eaten in small amounts. Chili, which is more Southwestern than Mexican, defies its "greasy-spoon" reputation; even a large bowl of chili has only 300 calories and twelve grams of fat (about thirty percent). Beans are one of the best sources of fiber, making chili with beans a great choice.

Breakfast: Simpler is Better

Making healthy choices for lunch or dinner may be easier than making them for breakfast. Generally, simpler is better when it comes to fast food breakfast foods. Start your day with plain muffins, biscuits, or toast. Pancakes are another surprisingly good option. Here's an example of the difference your fast food breakfast choices can make:

Breakfast 1

Sausage and egg biscuit,
hash brown potatoes,
large orange juice

820 calories

49 grams of fat

1475 milligrams of sodium

Breakfast 2

Scrambled egg, English muffin

366 calories

17 grams of fat

575 milligrams of sodium

Since many of us are eating fast food quite frequently, it's important that we learn how to do it healthfully. You can eat fast food and fit it into your meal plan, if you follow your good judgment about which fast foods you eat and how often you eat them. The chart below summarizes some options that you may face in any given restaurant. The right-hand column gives the recommended choice.

Instead of . . .

Deluxe burger
700 calories, 47 fat grams

Deep fried, breaded chicken
sandwich
500 calories, 25 fat grams

Super-stuffed baked potato
610 calories, 24 fat grams

Deluxe pizza, 2 slices
618 calories, 28 fat grams

Taco salad
580 calories, 30 fat grams

Giant muffin
705 calories, 30 fat grams

Heath Blizzard®
800 calories, 24 fat grams

Choose . . .

Hamburger
270 calories, 9 fat grams

Grilled chicken sandwich
300 calories, 14 fat grams

Plain baked potato
310 calories, 0 fat grams

Cheese pizza, 2 slices
344 calories, 10 fat grams

Grilled chicken salad,
low-calorie dressing
240 calories, 8 fat grams

Small muffin
158 calories, 4 fat grams

Soft serve cone
230 calories, 7 fat grams

FAST FOOD LIST

Food	Quantity	Calories	Fat (grams)	Carbohydrate Choices	Exchanges
Arby's®					
Chicken breast sandwich	1 sandwich	445	23	3½	3½ starch, 2 med. fat meat, 2 fat
French dip sub	1 sandwich	467	21	3	3 starch, 3 med. fat meat, 1 fat
Hot ham 'n cheese sandwich	1 sandwich	292	14	1	1 starch, 3 med. fat meat
Junior roast beef sandwich	1 sandwich	233	11	1½	1½ starch, 1 med. fat meat, 1 fat
Regular roast beef sandwich	1 sandwich	383	18	2	2 starch, 2 med. fat meat, 1 fat
Accompaniments					
Baked potato, plain	1 potato	290	1	4	4 starch
Garden salad, low-calorie Italian dressing	1 salad	57	1	½	2 veg
Potato cakes	1 cake	204	12	1	1 starch, 2 fat
Boston Market®					
White meat chicken (¼), corn bread, steamed vegetables, fruit salad	1 meal	502	12	4	3 starch, 1 fruit, 1 veg, 4 lean meat
White meat chicken without skin or wing	¼ chicken	164	4	0	4 very lean meat
Chicken breast sandwich	1 sandwich	422	4	3	3 starch, 5 very lean meat
Chicken soup	1 cup	87	3	0	1 veg, 1 lean meat
Accompaniments					
BBQ baked beans	1 order	290	7	3	3 starch, 1 fat
Buttered corn	1 order	181	6	2	2 starch, 1 fat
Corn bread	1 order	253	8	3	3 starch, 1 fat

Food	Quantity	Calories	Fat (grams)	Carbohydrate Choices	Exchanges
Macaroni and cheese	1 cup	290	11	2	2 starch, 1 med. fat meat, 1 fat
Mashed potatoes and gravy	1 order	205	10	2	2 starch, 2 fat
New potatoes	1 order	129	3	1½	1½ starch
Stuffing	1 order	282	11	2½	2½ starch, 2 fat

Desserts

Food	Quantity	Calories	Fat (grams)	Carbohydrate Choices	Exchanges
Chocolate chip cookie	1 (3 oz)	369	16	3	3 other carb, 3 fat

Burger King®

Food	Quantity	Calories	Fat (grams)	Carbohydrate Choices	Exchanges
BK Broiler®	1 sandwich	540	29	3	3 starch, 3 med. fat meat, 3 fat
Cheeseburger	1 sandwich	300	14	2	2 starch, 2 med. fat meat, 1 fat
Chicken Tenders® with BBQ sauce	6 pieces	250	12	1	1 starch, 2 med. fat meat
Hamburger	1 sandwich	260	10	2	2 starch, 2 med. fat meat
Whopper Jr.®	1 sandwich	410	21	2	2 starch, 2 med. fat meat, 3 fat

Accompaniments

Food	Quantity	Calories	Fat (grams)	Carbohydrate Choices	Exchanges
French fries	medium	400	20	3	3 starch, 4 fat
Garden salad, no dressing	1 salad	90	5	0	1 veg, 1 fat
Onion rings	1 order	310	15	3	3 starch, 3 fat

Dairy Queen®

Food	Quantity	Calories	Fat (grams)	Carbohydrate Choices	Exchanges
BBQ beef sandwich	1 sandwich	225	4	2	2 starch, 2 lean meat
Fish fillet sandwich	1 sandwich	370	16	2½	2½ starch, 2 med. fat meat, 1 fat
Grilled chicken sandwich	1 sandwich	300	8	2	2 starch, 3 lean meat
Hamburger	1 sandwich	310	13	2	2 starch, 2 med. fat meat, 1 fat

Food	Quantity	Calories	Fat (grams)	Carbohydrate Choices	Exchanges
Hot dog	1 sandwich	280	16	1½	1½ starch, 1 med. fat meat, 2 fat
Accompaniments					
French fries	small	210	10	2	2 starch, 2 fat
Desserts					
Dilly Bar®	1 bar	210	13	1½	1½ other carb, 2 fat
DQ Sandwich®	1 sandwich	140	4	1½	1½ other carb, 1 fat
Vanilla ice cream cone	regular	230	7	2½	2½ other carb, 1 fat
Yogurt cone	regular	180	<1	2½	2½ other carb

Domino's Pizza

Food	Quantity	Calories	Fat (grams)	Carbohydrate Choices	Exchanges
Hand-Tossed Pizza					
Cheese, 12"	2 slices	344	10	3	3 starch, 2 med. fat meat
Ham, 12"	2 slices	362	10	3	3 starch, 2 med. fat meat
Thin Crust Pizza					
Cheese, 12"	½ pizza	364	16	3	3 starch, 1 med. fat meat, 2 fat
Pepperoni, 12"	½ pizza	447	23	3	3 starch, 2 med. fat meat, 3 fat
Deep Dish Pizza					
Cheese, 12"	2 slices	560	24	4	4 starch, 2 med. fat meat, 3 fat
Italian sausage and mushroom, 12"	2 slices	618	28	4	4 starch, 1 veg, 2 med. fat meat, 4 fat

Hardee's®

Food	Quantity	Calories	Fat (grams)	Carbohydrate Choices	Exchanges
Chef salad	1 salad	200	14	½	1 veg, 3 med. fat meat
Chicken fillet sandwich	1 sandwich	400	14	3	3 starch, 2 med. fat meat, 1 fat
Hamburger	1 sandwich	260	9	2	2 starch, 1 med. fat meat, 1 fat

Food	Quantity	Calories	Fat (grams)	Carbohydrate Choices	Exchanges
Roast beef sandwich, regular	1 sandwich	270	11	2	2 starch, 2 med. fat meat
Accompaniments					
French fries	medium	350	15	3	3 starch, 3 fat
Side salad	1 salad	20	1	0	1 veg
Desserts					
Cool Twist® vanilla or chocolate cone	1 cone	180	4	2	2 other carb, 1 fat
KFC®					
Original Recipe					
Chicken breast	1 piece	360	20	1	1 starch, 4 med. fat meat
Chicken drumstick	1 piece	130	7	0	2 med. fat meat
Extra Tasty Crispy					
Chicken breast	1 piece	470	28	2	2 starch, 4 med. fat meat, 2 fat
Chicken drumstick	1 piece	190	11	½	½ starch, 2 med. fat meat
Accompaniments					
Cole slaw	1 small	114	6	½	2 veg, 1 fat
Corn-on-the-cob	1 medium	222	12	2	2 starch, 2 fat
Mashed potatoes with gravy	1 small	109	5	1	1 starch, 1 fat
Long John Silver's®					
Baked chicken, rice, green beans, slaw, roll	1 entrée	590	15	5	5 starch, 1 veg, 3 med. fat meat
Baked fish with lemon crumb, rice, green beans, slaw, roll	3-piece dinner	610	13	5	5 starch, 2 veg, 4 lean meat
Fish and fries	2-piece dinner	610	37	3½	3½ starch, 3 med. fat meat, 4 fat
Light portion fish with lemon crumb, rice, side salad	2-piece dinner	330	5	3	3 starch, 1 veg, 3 very lean meat

Food	Quantity	Calories	Fat (grams)	Carbohydrate Choices	Exchanges
McDonald's®					
Arch Deluxe™	1 sandwich	550	31	2½	2½ starch, 3 med. fat meat, 3 fat
Arch Deluxe with Bacon™	1 sandwich	590	34	2½	2½ starch, 4 med. fat meat, 3 fat
Big Mac®	1 sandwich	560	31	3	3 starch, 3 med. fat meat, 3 fat
Cheeseburger	1 sandwich	320	13	2	2 starch, 1½ med. fat meat, 1 fat
Chef salad	1 salad	210	11	½	2 veg, 2 med. fat meat
Chicken McNuggets®	6 pieces	300	18	1	1 starch, 2 med. fat meat, 1 fat
Crispy Chicken Deluxe™	1 sandwich	500	25	3	3 starch, 3 med. fat meat, 2 fat
Fish Fillet Deluxe™	1 sandwich	560	28	3½	3½ starch, 2½ med. fat meat, 3 fat
Grilled Chicken Deluxe™	1 sandwich	440	20	2½	2½ starch, 3 med. fat meat, 1 fat
Hamburger	1 sandwich	260	9	2	2 starch, 1½ med. fat meat
Quarter Pounder®	1 sandwich	420	21	2½	2½ starch, 3 med. fat meat, 1 fat
Quarter Pounder® with Cheese	1 sandwich	530	30	2½	2½ starch, 3½ med. fat meat, 1 fat
Accompaniments					
French fries	medium	320	17	2½	2½ starch, 3 fat
Garden salad	1 salad	80	4	0	1 veg
Lite vinaigrette dressing	2 oz pkt	48	2	½	½ other carb
Syrup	1 pkt	190	<1	3	3 other carb

Food	Quantity	Calories	Fat (grams)	Carbohydrate Choices	Exchanges
Breakfast Items					
Egg McMuffin®	1 sandwich	290	13	3	3 starch, 2 med. fat meat
English muffin with butter	1 muffin	170	5	2	2 starch, 1 fat
Hot cakes (plain)	1 order	280	4	3½	3½ starch, 1 fat
Scrambled eggs	1 order	170	12	0	2 med. fat meat
Desserts					
Vanilla reduced-fat ice cream cone	1 cone	150	5	1½	1½ other carb
Pizza Hut®					
Hand-Tossed Pizza					
Cheese	1 slice	235	7	2	2 starch, 1 med. fat meat
Supreme	1 slice	284	12	2	2 starch, 2 med. fat meat
Pan Pizza					
Cheese	1 slice	261	11	2	2 starch, 1 med. fat meat, 1 fat
Supreme	1 slice	311	15	2	2 starch, 2 med. fat meat, 1 fat
Personal Pan Pizza					
Pepperoni	1 pizza	637	28	4½	4½ starch, 2 med. fat meat, 4 fat
Supreme	1 pizza	722	34	5	5 starch, 3 med. fat meat, 4 fat
Thin 'N Crispy Pizza					
Cheese	1 slice	205	8	1½	1½ starch, 1 med. fat meat, 1 fat
Supreme	1 slice	257	13	1½	1½ starch, 1 med. fat meat, 2 fat

Food	Quantity	Calories	Fat (grams)	Carbohydrate Choices	Exchanges
Red Lobster®					
Broiled fish sandwich	4 oz	300	10	2	2 starch, 3 lean meat
Crab legs	16 oz	120	1	0	4 very lean meat
Grilled chicken breast	4 oz	170	6	0	3 lean meat
Today's Fresh Catch	5 oz	165	6	0	4 lean meat
Accompaniments					
Baked potato	8 oz	270	trace	3	3 starch
Cocktail sauce	1 oz	30	0	½	1 veg
Rice pilaf	4 oz	140	3	1½	1½ starch, 1 fat
Shrimp cocktail	6 large	90	2	0	2 very lean meat
Subway®					
Cold Cut Combo sub	6" sub	427	20	3	3 starch, 2 med. fat meat, 2 fat
Meatball sub	6" sub	459	22	3	3 starch, 2 med. fat meat, 2 fat
Roast beef sub	6" sub	345	12	3	3 starch, 2 med. fat meat
Turkey breast sub	6" sub	322	10	3	3 starch, 2 med. fat meat
Taco Bell®					
Bean burrito	1 burrito	391	12	4	4 starch, 1 med. fat meat, 1 fat
Beef burrito	1 burrito	432	19	3	3 starch, 2 med. fat meat, 2 fat
Soft taco	1 taco	223	11	1	1 starch, 1 med. fat meat, 1 fat
Taco	1 taco	180	11	1	1 starch, 1 med. fat meat
Taco salad	1 salad	838	55	3½	3½ starch, 1 veg, 3 med. fat meat, 8 fat

Food	Quantity	Calories	Fat (grams)	Carbohydrate Choices	Exchanges
Taco salad, light	1 salad	680	25	5	5 starch, 1 veg, 3 med. fat meat, 2 fat
Tostada	1 tostada	242	11	2	2 starch, 1 med. fat meat, 1 fat
Wendy's®					
Breaded chicken sandwich	1 sandwich	450	20	3	3 starch, 3 med. fat meat, 1 fat
Chili	1 bowl (12 oz)	290	9	2	2 starch, 3 lean
Grilled chicken sandwich	1 sandwich	290	7	2	2 starch, 3 lean meat
Hamburger, single, plain	1 sandwich	350	15	2	2 starch, 3 med. fat meat
Taco salad	1 salad	640	30	3	3 starch, 3 med. fat meat, 3 fat
Accompaniments					
Baked potato, plain	1 potato	310	<1	4	4 starch
Deluxe garden salad	1 salad	110	5	½	2 veg, 1 fat
Reduced-calorie Italian dressing	2 Tbsp	50	4	0	1 fat
Sour cream	1 pkt	60	6	0	1 fat
Desserts					
Chocolate chip cookie	1 cookie	270	11	2½	2½ other carb, 2 fat
White Castle®					
Hamburger	2 small	322	16	2	2 starch, 1 med. fat meat, 2 fat
Accompaniments					
French fries	1 order	301	15	2½	2½ starch, 3 fat

CHAPTER 25

Exchanges for Convenience Foods

If nutrition is an important factor in our food choices, so too is convenience. When we're not grabbing a bite at a fast food restaurant, we're looking for a home-cooked meal that's easy to prepare so we can spend time on other pursuits. Convenience foods, such as frozen dinners and boxed rice and pasta mixes, are the fastest growing processed food group today. Convenience foods give us what we demand—quick, easy-to-prepare, good-tasting, and relatively inexpensive meals. Fortunately, balancing convenience with good nutrition is not hard to do, as long as you keep a few simple guidelines in mind.

The biggest problems associated with convenience foods are too much fat, too much saturated fat, and too much sodium. However, the many low-fat food products now available have made it easier to find foods that fit easily into a healthy meal plan. Moreover, the Nutrition Facts panel found on every packaged food item gives you information about calories, fat, saturated fat, sodium, and other nutrients. Try to choose foods that meet the following nutrition guidelines.

Type of Food	Fat	Sodium
Meals and entrées (frozen dinners, frozen pizza, etc.)	3 grams or less per 100 calories	No more than 800 milligrams per meal or entrée
Cheese	5 grams or less per serving	No more than 400 milligrams per ounce
Side dishes, snacks, cereals and other foods	3 grams or less per 15 grams of carbohydrate	No more than 400 milligrams per serving
Processed meats	3 grams or less per ounce	No more than 400 milligrams per ounce

CONVENIENCE FOOD LIST

Food	Quantity	Carbohydrate Choices	Exchanges
Frozen Dinners			
Dinners, 8 oz	1 dinner	2	2 starch, 1–2 med. fat meat
Dinners, 11 oz	1 dinner	2	2 starch, 1 veg, 2–3 med. fat meat, 1–2 fat
Dinners, 16 oz	1 dinner	3	3 starch, 1 veg, 3 med. fat meat, 2–3 fat
Dinners with less than 300 calories, 11 oz	1 dinner	2	2 starch, 1 veg, 1–2 lean meat
Healthy Choice® dinners, 11 oz	1 dinner	2	2 starch, 1 veg, 2 lean meat
Mexican dinners, 11 oz	1 dinner	3½	3½ starch, 1 med. fat meat, 1 fat
Oriental dinners, 9 oz	1 dinner	2	2 starch, 1 veg, 1–2 lean meat
Frozen Entrées			
Burrito	1 (5 oz)	3	3 starch, 1 med. fat meat, 1 fat
Chili with beans	1 cup	1–2	1–2 starch, 2 med. fat meat, 0–1 fat
Family-size entrées	1 cup	2	2 starch, 1–2 med. fat meat
French bread pizza	1 pizza	3	3 starch, 2 med. fat meat, 1 fat
Hamburger Helper®	1 cup	2	2 starch, 2–3 med. fat meat, 1 fat
Hot Pockets®	1 sandwich	2½	2½ starch, 1–2 med. fat meat, 1 fat
Lasagna	1 cup	2	2 starch, 1–2 med. fat meat, 0–1 fat

Food	Quantity	Carbohydrate Choices	Exchanges
Lunch Bucket®	1 bucket (8½ oz)	2	1–2 starch, 1 med. fat meat
Lunch Express® entrées	1 entrée (9 oz)	2½	2½ starch, 1–2 med. fat meat
Lunchables®, meat and cheese	1 pkg (4.5 oz)	22	1½ 1½ starch, 3 med. fat meat, 1 fat
Macaroni and cheese	1 cup	2	2 starch, 1 med. fat meat, 1 fat
Microcup entrées	1 entrée (7.5 oz)	2	1–2 starch, 1–2 med. fat meat, 1 fat
Oriental entrées	1 entrée (13 oz)	4	3–4 starch, 1 lean meat
Oriental light entrées	1 entrée (11.25 oz)	3	2–3 starch, 1 veg, 1 lean meat
Pasta Classics®	1 entrée (12 oz)	3	3 starch, 1 veg, 2 lean meat
Pizza, 10"	¼ pizza	2	2 starch, 2 med. fat meat, 1–2 fat
Pot pie	1 pie (7 oz)	2	2 starch, 1 veg, 1 med. fat meat, 3–4 fat
Spaghetti dinner, canned	1 cup	2–3	2–3 starch, 1 med. fat meat, 0–1 fat
Tuna Helper®	1 cup	2	2 starch, 1–2 med. fat meat

Side Dishes

Food	Quantity	Carbohydrate Choices	Exchanges
Noodles romanoff	½ cup	1	1 starch, 1 med. fat meat, 1 fat
Potatoes, au gratin	½ cup	1½	1½ starch, 1 fat
Potato salad	½ cup	1	1 starch, 2 fat
Rice, fried with chicken and pork	1 cup	3	3 starch, 1 med. fat meat

Food	Quantity	Carbohydrate Choices	Exchanges
Scalloped potatoes	½ cup	1½	1½ starch, 1 fat
Stuffing mix, microwave	½ cup	1½	1½ starch, 1–2 fat
Suddenly Salad®	¾ cup	2	2 starch, 1–2 fat
Tater tots	3 small (3 oz)	1	1 starch, 1½ fat
Twice-baked potato	½ potato (5 oz)	2	2 starch, 2 fat

Breads

Food	Quantity	Carbohydrate Choices	Exchanges
Breadsticks, average	6 breadsticks	1	1 starch
Croissants	1 medium	1½	1½ starch, 3 fat
Croissants, petite	1 small	1	1 starch, 1½ fat
Dinner rolls	1 small	1	1 starch
Muffins	1 muffin	1½	1–1½ starch, 1 fat
Light	1 muffin	1½	1½ starch
Quick bread mixes	1⁄16 loaf	1	1 starch, 1 fat

Soups

Food	Quantity	Carbohydrate Choices	Exchanges
Bean	1 cup	1	1 starch, 1 very lean meat
Chunky® Soups	1 can (10¾ oz)	1½	1 starch, 1 veg, 1 med. fat meat
Cream soups (made with water)	1 cup	1½	1½ starch, 1 fat
Cup-A-Soup®, broth-type	1 envelope (6 oz)	0	free
Cup-A-Soup®, creamy	1 envelope (6 oz)	1	1 starch
Cup O' Noodles®	1 container	2	2 starch, 3 fat
Microcup Hearty	1 container (7.5 oz)	1	1 starch, 1 lean meat
Ramen noodles	½ pkg (1½ oz)	2	2 starch, 1½ fat
Low-fat	½ pkg (1½ oz)	3	3 starch
Split pea (made with water)	1 cup	2	2 starch
Tomato, vegetable beef, chicken noodle, or other broth-type	1 cup	1	1 starch

Breakfast Items

Food	Quantity	Carbohydrate Choices	Exchanges
Egg Beaters®	½ cup	0	1 lean meat
French toast, frozen	1 slice	1	1 starch, ½ med. fat meat

Food	Quantity	Carbohydrate Choices	Exchanges
Pancakes (as prepared from mix)	3 cakes (4" across)	2	2 starch, 1 fat
Microwave, 3½" across	2 cakes	1	1 starch, 1 fat
Waffles, frozen, 4½" square	1 waffle	1	1 starch, 1 fat

Desserts

Food	Quantity	Carbohydrate Choices	Exchanges
Almost Home® cookies, all varieties	2 cookies (2 oz)	1	1 starch, 1 fat
American Collection® cookies, all varieties	1 cookie	1	1 other carb, 1 fat
Cake, fat-free	1 slice (1 oz)	1	1 other carb
Frozen dairy dessert	4 oz	1½	1½ other carb
Gingersnaps	3 cookies	1	1 other carb
Kitchen Hearth® cookies	3 cookies	1	1 other carb, 1½ fat
Lovin' Lites® cake, all varieties	⅒ cake	2½	2½ other carb
Supermoist® cake, all varieties	⅟₁₂ cake	2	2 other carb, 2 fat

CHAPTER 26

Exchanges for Smart Snacking

Each year Americans crunch their way through over twenty-five billion dollars worth of snack foods. This is not necessarily a dire statistic—although snacking often has a bad name, snacks can add both nutritional value and enjoyment to a meal plan. Even if you're trying to lose weight, consider snacks your friend; by helping to satisfy your hunger throughout the day, they can help you avoid overeating at meal times. But if you're not careful, snacks can contribute a significant amount of fat, salt, and calories to your diet. It pays to select your snack foods wisely.

Try to select snacks that provide solid nutrition and are low in fat, calories, and salt. Fruits and vegetables, nonfat plain and artificially-sweetened yogurt, and whole-grain breads and muffins all provide important nutrients. On packaged snack foods, let the Nutrition Facts panel be your guide. Look for snack foods that contain three grams or less fat and 400 milligrams or less sodium per serving. Finding chips, cookies, and other foods that meet these guidelines is easier than it used to be, given the low-fat and fat-free items that now flood supermarket shelves. These reduced-fat items are good options, but use them cautiously—they still supply calories, and the low-fat label can tempt you into eating more than the recommended serving size.

Tips for Smart Snacking

- Choose high-fiber snacks that will help you feel full. Some good examples are fruits and vegetables, whole-grain toast or muffins, or baked tortilla chips with bean dip.
- Avoid keeping high-fat, high-calorie snacks around the house or workplace; if they're not available, you can't eat them.

- Season snacks with spices such as garlic or onion powder, dill, basil, or lemon juice instead of salt.
- Beware of commercially manufactured snack bars or "energy bars." Most are similar to candy bars and are scarcely more than fat, sugar, and salt with a little flavoring.
- If your meal plan includes snacks, don't skip them. Use a snack that fits into your number of food exchanges, and watch the portion size.
- Remember, "fat free" and "sugar free" do not necessarily mean "calorie free" or even "low calorie." Read the Nutrition Facts panel on the package or label to get accurate nutrition information about foods.

If you have diabetes, snacks are an important part of your meal plan. Snacks help distribute your carbohydrate intake throughout the day. If you eat too much carbohydrate at one time, your blood glucose levels can go too high. Snacks also help prevent blood glucose levels from dropping too low between meals; they are especially important for people taking insulin.

The times when you may need a snack depend on your insulin regimen (if any), your age, your activity level, and your calorie needs. In general, children using injected insulin do well with a mid-morning, a mid-afternoon, and a bedtime snack. Some children do even better with two afternoon snacks, depending on the times of their school lunch and their dinner. Adults often need an afternoon and an evening snack.

In addition to knowing when to snack, you also need to know what and how much to eat. Eating too much of even a healthy snack can contribute more calories than you need and can cause blood glucose levels to soar. The following are ideas for healthy snacks:

- Bread or toast (whole grain), bagels, English muffins, or breadsticks
- Cereal snack mix (prepare with garlic powder, Worcestershire sauce, and a small amount of margarine)
- Cookies made with whole grains, oil, and minimal sugar
- Commercial cookies such as animal crackers, gingersnaps, fig bars, and molasses cookies
- Low-fat or nonfat crackers (graham, melba, matzo, oyster crackers)

- Low-fat frozen yogurt
- Frozen fruit or yogurt bars
- Fruit (canned, dried, or fresh)
- Nonfat plain or artificially-sweetened fruit yogurt
- Popcorn (air-popped or microwave light, served plain, lightly salted, or sprinkled with Parmesan cheese)
- Pretzels
- Tortilla chips (baked, not fried) with salsa
- Trail mix (popcorn, raisins, peanuts, and dried fruits)
- Vegetables (raw, cooked, or served with low-fat dips)
- Fruit and nut breads

Sometimes the best and healthiest snack choice just isn't convenient. We often have to weigh the ideal against what's practical at any given time. When convenience wins out, the following "legal junk foods" can help you choose the best from what's available.

SNACK FOOD LIST

Food	Quantity	Fat (grams)	Carbohydrate Choices	Exchanges
Beverages				
Apple cider	½ cup	0	1	1 fruit
All Sport® Thirst Quencher	1 cup (8 oz)	0	1	1 other carb
Carnation® hot cocoa	1 pkt	1	1½	1½ other carb
Fat free	1 pkt	0	0	free
No sugar added	1 pkt	0	½	½ other carb
Catawba juice	¾ cup	0	1	1 fruit
Chocolate milk	1 cup (8 oz)	1.5	2	2 other carb
Cocoa mix, hot, sugar free	1 envelope (6 oz)	0	½	½ other carb
Cranberry juice	⅓ cup	0	1	1 fruit
Cranberry juice or cranapple drink, low-calorie	1 cup	0	1	1 fruit or 1 other carb
Fruit juice, canned	1 can (6 oz)	0	1½	1½ fruit

Food	Quantity	Fat (grams)	Carbohydrate Choices	Exchanges
Fruit nectars (apricot, peach, pear)	⅓ cup	0	1	1 fruit
Gatorade®	1 cup (8 oz)	0	1	1 other carb
Hawaiian Punch®, low-calorie	1 cup	0	1	1 other carb
Powerade®	1 cup (8 oz)	0	1	1 other carb
Sundance® sparkling beverage	1 bottle (5 oz)	0	1	1 other carb
Swiss Miss® hot cocoa, fat-free	1 pkt	0	½	½ other carb
Light	1 pkt	0.5	1	1 other carb
No sugar added	1 pkt	0	1	1 other carb
Tang®	1 cup (8 oz)	0	1½	1½ other carb
Sugar-free	1 cup (8 oz)	0	free	free
Tomato juice, vegetable juice cocktail	1½ cup	1	1	1 fruit
V8® juice	1 can (5.5 oz)	0	½	1 veg

Chips/Pretzels/Popcorn, etc.

Food	Quantity	Fat (grams)	Carbohydrate Choices	Exchanges
Bugles®, 50% less fat	1½ cups	3.5	1½	1½ starch, 1 fat
Caramel corn	½ cup (1 oz)	2.5	2	2 starch
Fat-free	¾ cup	0	1½	1½ starch
Caramel puff corn	¾ cup	2	1½	1½ starch
Cheese puffs	25 puffs (1 oz)	11	1	1 starch, 2 fat
Cheetos®	1 oz	10	1	1 starch, 2 fat
Chex® Snack Mix	⅔ cup	3.5	1	1 starch, 1 fat
Combos®, cheddar cheese	⅓ cup	5	1	1 starch, 1 fat
Corn chips, all varieties	34 chips	9	1	1 starch, 2 fat
Cracker Jack® popcorn	½ cup	4.5	1½	1½ starch, 1 fat
Doritos® corn chips, all varieties	~34 chips (1 oz)	7	1	1 starch, 1 fat
Fritos® corn chips, all varieties	~34 chips (1 oz)	10	1	1 starch, 2 fat
Guiltless Gourmet® tortilla chips	1 oz	1	1½	1½ starch
Oriental rice cracker mix	½ cup	0	1½	1½ starch
Party mix	⅓ cup (1 oz)	5	1	1 starch, 1 fat

Food	Quantity	Fat (grams)	Carbohydrate Choices	Exchanges
Popcorn				
Air popped	5 cups	0	1	1 starch
Cheese-flavored	3 cups (1 oz)	9	1	1 starch, 2 fat
Fat-free	3 cups (1 oz)	0	1	1 starch
Light	5 cups	2.5	1	1 starch, ½ fat
Microwave, with butter	5 cups	10	1	1 starch, 2 fat
Popcorn bar	1 bar	1	1	1 starch
Popcorn cake	2 cakes	1	1	1 starch
Mini	8 cakes	1	1	1 starch
Potato chips	12–18 chips (1 oz)	10	1	1 starch, 2 fat
Baked, low-fat	12–18 chips (1 oz)	2.5	1½	1½ starch, ½ fat
Fat-free	12–18 chips (1 oz)	0	1½	1½ starch
Reduced fat	12–18 chips (1 oz)	6.5	1	1 starch, 1 fat
Pretzels	1 oz	0	1½	1½ starch
Sticks, very thin	65 sticks	0	1	1 starch
Twists	4 twists	1	0	1 starch
Rice cakes, 4" across	2 cakes	0	1	1 starch
Mini	½ oz	0	1	1 starch
Sesame sticks	¼ cup (1 oz)	10	1	1 starch, 2 fat
Snack cracker mix	⅓ cup (1 oz)	4.5	1	1 starch, 1 fat
Snack mix	½ cup	8	1½	1½ starch, 1 fat
Reduced fat	½ cup	4.5	1½	1½ starch, 1 fat
Sun Chips®	1 oz	6	1	1 starch, 1 fat
Tortilla chips, fried	15–18 chips (1 oz)	6	1	1 starch, 1 fat
Baked	15–18 chips (1 oz)	1	1½	1½ starch
Trail mix with raisin, nuts, coconut, and dried fruit	¼ cup	8	1	1 starch, 1 fat
Tropical	¼ cup	5	1	1 starch, 1 fat
With chocolate chips	¼ cup	9	1	1 starch, 2 fat
Yogurt-covered pretzels	7 (1 oz)	6	1½	1½ starch, 1 fat

Food	Quantity	Fat (grams)	Carbohydrate Choices	Exchanges
Cookies				
Animal crackers	8 cookies	2	1	1 other carb
Archway® cookies, fat-free	1 cookie (1 oz)	0	1½	1½ other carb
Chips Ahoy®	3 cookies	8	1½	1½ other carb, 1½ fat
Reduced fat	3 cookies	6	1½	1½ other carb, 1 fat
Cookies, average	1 cookie (3" across)	5	1	1 other carb, 1 fat
Dinosaur cookies, mini	14 cookies	3.5	1	1 other carb, ½ fat
Fig Newtons® or fig bars	2 cookies	0	1½	1½ other carb
Frookie®, apple cobbler	1 cookie	0	1	1 other carb or 1 fruit
Frookie®, animal frackers	14 cookies	5	1	1 other carb, 1 fat
Gingersnaps	3 cookies	2	1	1 other carb
Fudge Stripe®, reduced-fat	3 cookies	4.5	1	1 other carb, 1 fat
Health Valley® jumbo fruit cookie	1 cookie	0	1	1 other carb
Koala yummies	13 cookies	10	1	1 other carb, 2 fat
Lorna Doone® shortbread	6 cookies	7	1	1 other carb, 1 fat
Oatmeal raisin cookies	2 cookies	7	1	1 other carb, 1 fat
Pepperidge Farm® soft-baked reduced-fat chocolate chunk	1 cookie	3	1	1 other carb
Salerno® butter cookies	6 cookies	7	1½	1½ other carb, 1 fat
Reduced fat	6 cookies	5	1½	1½ other carb, 1 fat
Mini	25 cookies	6	1	1 other carb, 1 fat
Snackwell's® bite-size chocolate chip	13 cookies	3.5	1½	1½ other carb, ½ fat
Snackwell's® cinnamon graham snacks	20 cookies	0	2	2 other carb
Snackwell's® double fudge	1 cookie	0	1	1 other carb

Food	Quantity	Fat (grams)	Carbohydrate Choices	Exchanges
Sunshine® oatmeal cookie	3 cookies	7	1½	1½ other carb, 1 fat
Teddy Grahams®	25 cookies	4	1½	1½ other carb, 1 fat
Vanilla wafers	8 cookies	6	1½	1½ other carb, 1 fat
Reduced fat	8 cookies	2	1½	1½ other carb

Crackers

Food	Quantity	Fat (grams)	Carbohydrate Choices	Exchanges
Breadsticks, 4" long x ¼" thick	6 breadsticks	1	1	1 starch
Breton® wafers	6 crackers	6	1	1 starch, 1 fat
Reduced fat	6 crackers	3	1	1 starch, ½ fat
Cheese Nips®	20 crackers	6	1	1 starch, 1 fat
Reduced fat	22 crackers	3.5	1½	1½ starch, ½ fat
Cheez 'n Crackers®	1 package	7	½	½ starch, ½ med. fat meat, 1 fat
Chicken in a Biskit®	14 crackers (1 oz)	9	1	1 starch, 2 fat
Cracker sandwiches, reduced-fat	1 oz	7	1½	1½ starch, 1 fat
Garden Crisps®, vegetable	11 crackers	3	1	1 starch, ½ fat
Goldfish® crackers	45 crackers	6	1	1 starch, 1 fat
Grahams, cinnamon crisp, or chocolate	1 square (1 oz)	5	1½	1½ starch, 1 fat
Grahams, honey	1 square (1 oz)	6	1½	1½ starch, 1 fat
Harvest Crisps®, 5-Grain & Oat	12 crackers	5	1	1 starch, 1 fat
Hi-Ho® crackers	6 crackers	8	1	1 starch, 1 fat
Melba toast, long	4 slices	0	1	1 starch
Melba toast, rounds	8 crackers	0	1	1 starch
Oyster crackers	24 large or 42 small	0	1	1 starch
Peanut Butter 'N Cheez®	1 package	9	1	1 starch, ½ med. fat meat, 1 fat
Ritz®	6 crackers	4	1	1 starch, 1 fat
Ritz® Bits	40 crackers	5	1	1 starch, 1 fat
RyKrisp®	3 crackers	0	1	1 starch
Snackwell's® snack crackers	32 crackers	2	1½	1½ starch

Food	Quantity	Fat (grams)	Carbohydrate Choices	Exchanges
Snackwell's® wheat crackers	5 crackers	0	1	1 starch
Sociables® flavor crisps	8 crackers	4	1	1 starch, 1 fat
Triscuits®	6 crackers	5	1	1 starch, 1 fat
Vegetable Thins®	18 crackers	4	1½	1½ starch, 1 fat
Wasa® Bread crackers	2 slices	1	1	1 starch
Wheat Thins®	18 crackers	4	1½	1½ starch, 1 fat
Wheatables®	24 crackers	7	1	1 starch, 1 fat

Fruit Snacks

Food	Quantity	Fat (grams)	Carbohydrate Choices	Exchanges
Applesauce, natural	½ cup	0	1	1 fruit
Dried fruit	¼ cup (½ oz)	0	1	1 fruit
Fruit bar	1 bar	0	1	1 other carb
Fruit cup	½ cup	0	1	1 fruit
Fruit by the Foot®	1 roll	1	1	1 other carb
Fun Fruit®	1 pouch	0	1½	1½ other carb
Fruit juice bar, 100% juice	1 bar	0.5	1	1 other carb
Fruit Roll-Up®	1 (½ oz)	1	1	1 other carb
Fruit Wrinkle®	1 pouch	0	1½	1½ other carb
Mama Tish's® Italian Ice	½ cup	0	1½	1½ other carb
Nutty banana	⅔ cup	16	1½	1½ fruit, 3 fat
Raisins	½ oz box	0	1	1 fruit

Granola/Cereal Bars

Food	Quantity	Fat (grams)	Carbohydrate Choices	Exchanges
Breakfast bar	1 bar	6	1½	1½ other carb, 1 fat
Fudge-dipped granola bar	1 bar	3	1½	1½ other carb, ½ fat
Health Valley® bar	1 bar	0	2	2 other carb
Nature Valley® low-fat chewy granola bar	1 bar	2	1½	1½ other carb
Nutri-Grain® bar	1 bar	3	2½	2½ other carb, ½ fat
Snackwell's® cereal bar	1 bar	0	2	2 other carb
Toaster pastry	1 pastry	1	2½	2½ other carb

Food	Quantity	Fat (grams)	Carbohydrate Choices	Exchanges
Ice Cream/Frozen Snacks				
Ben & Jerry's® ice cream	½ cup	17	1½	1½ other carb, 3 fat
Breyers® ice cream	½ cup	8	1	1 other carb, 1½ fat
Fat-free	½ cup	0	1½	1½ other carb
Light	½ cup	4.5	1	1 other carb, 1 fat
No sugar added	½ cup	4	1	1 other carb, 1 fat
Breyers® low-fat frozen yogurt	½ cup	2.5	1½	1½ other carb
Colombo® nonfat frozen yogurt	½ cup	0	1½	1½ other carb
Dairy Queen® cone	1 small	5	1½	1½ other carb, 1 fat
Dannon® light frozen yogurt	½ cup	0	1½	1½ other carb
Dole® fruit & juice bar	1 bar	0	1	1 other carb
Dove® Bar, dark chocolate	1 bar	17	1½	1½ other carb, 3 fat
DQ® sandwich	1 sandwich	4	1½	1½ other carb, 1 fat
Eskimo Pie®	1 pie	11	1	1 other carb, 2 fat
No sugar added	1 pie	11	1	1 other carb, 2 fat
Reduced fat	1 pie	8	1	1 other carb, 1½ fat
Fruit ice	½ cup	0	1	1 other carb
Fudgesicle®, no sugar added	1 bar	0.5	½	½ other carb
Haagen Dazs® ice cream	½ cup	18	1½	1½ other carb, 3 fat
Fat-free sorbet	½ cup	0	2	2 other carb
Fat-free sorbet bar	1 bar	0	1	1 other carb
Popsicle®	1 bar	0	1	1 other carb
Sugar-free	1 bar	0	0	free
Push-Up®	1 bar	2	1	1 other carb
Snackwell's® low-fat ice cream sandwich	1 sandwich	1.5	1	1 other carb
Yoplait® nonfat frozen yogurt bar	1 bar	0	1	1 other carb

Food	Quantity	Fat (grams)	Carbohydrate Choices	Exchanges
Meat and Related Snacks				
Beef jerky	½ oz	1	0	1 very lean meat
Buddig® meats	1 oz	2	0	1 lean meat
Cheez Whiz®	2 Tbsp	8	0	1 high fat meat
Cottage cheese, low-fat or nonfat	¼ cup	2.5	0	1 very lean meat
Nuts	¼ cup (1 oz)	16	0	1 med. fat meat, 2 fat
Nut mix	¼ cup (1 oz)	15	½	1 med. fat meat, 2 fat
Peanut butter	1 Tbsp	8	0	1 high fat meat
Pickled herring	1 oz	2	0	1 med. fat meat
Sardines	2 medium	3	0	1 lean meat
String cheese	1 oz	5	0	1 med. fat meat
Sunflower seeds	¼ cup (1 oz)	15	½	1 med. fat meat, 2 fat
Velveeta® slices or spread	1 slice or 1 oz	9	0	1 high fat meat
Snack Cakes/Bars/Pastries				
Hostess® cupcake, low-fat	1 (5 oz)	4	5	5 other carb
Kellogg's® Rice Crispy Treats®	1 bar	2	1	1 other carb
Muffins, fruit, fat-free, all varieties	1 small	0	2	1 starch, 1 fruit
Pop Tarts®, low-fat	1 tart	3	2½	2½ other carb
Sweet Rewards® bar	1 bar	0	2	2 other carb
Twinkies®, low-fat	1 cake	1.5	2	2 other carb
Soup				
Bouillon or beef broth	1 cup	0	0	free
Cup-A-Soup®, broth-type	6 oz	0	0	free
Cup-A-Soup®, cream-type	6 oz	2	1	1 starch
Cup-A-Soup®, Country Style	6 oz	1	1	1 starch

Food	Quantity	Fat (grams)	Carbohydrate Choices	Exchanges
Yogurt and Pudding				
Dannon® plain lowfat yogurt	1 cup (8 oz)	5	1	1 milk, 1 fat
Fruit on the bottom	1 cup (8 oz)	3	3	1 milk, 2 other carb
Light	1 cup (8 oz)	0	1	1 milk
Light and crunchy	1 cup (8 oz)	0	2	1 milk, 1 other carb
Gelatin snack cups	1 snack (4 oz)	0	1	1 other carb
Sugar-free	1 snack (4 oz)	0	0	free
Jell-O® sugar-free pudding	½ cup	0	1	1 milk or 1 other carb
Pudding cups	1 snack (4 oz)	5	1½	1½ other carb, 1 fat
Fat-free	1 snack (4 oz)	0	1½	1½ other carb
Yogurt sweetened with NutraSweet® or light yogurt	1 container	0	1	1 milk

CHAPTER 27

Exchanges for Camping

Camping is becoming more popular every year, because it gives people an opportunity to get away from busy, noisy lives and to enjoy nature at its purest. The amount of meal planning you need for camping depends on the type of camping you plan to do. When you camp with a motor home or camper trailer, you can take nearly any type of food because refrigeration and adequate storage areas are available. You can bring along food that is similar to what you eat at home.

Canoeing and backpacking require more careful planning. For canoeing, food must be compact, lightweight, and non-perishable in order to be carried on portages and packed into confined areas of the canoe. Weight is even more important in backpacking, because everything—sleeping bag, tent, cooking equipment, and food—must be carried on your back. But despite weight and space considerations, it's important to choose foods that are filling and nutritious (not just s'mores!).

Whatever type of camping you plan to do, be sure to pack enough food for the duration of the trip. It sounds obvious, but it's easy to underestimate the amount of food you'll need—people forget that increased exercise means an increased appetite. Experienced campers solve this problem by planning daily menus. Food for each day can then be packed separately and labeled with the date and time it is to be eaten. Bring slightly more food than you think you'll need, in case a pack is lost or damaged.

Freeze-dried and dehydrated foods are compact, convenient options for camping. Freeze-dried foods are best because their flavor is more like fresh foods and they are virtually foolproof in preparation—just add water and serve. When packaged in laminated aluminum foil and vacuum-sealed in plastic, they will last indefinitely. (Dehydrated foods must be discarded after one year.) You can usually purchase freeze-dried foods anywhere you can buy camping gear, and companies that manufacture these products (Alpine Aire, Mountain House, Richmoor Corporation, Natural High, Backpacker's Pantry) can supply nutrition analyses. See appendix 1 for more information.

If You Have Diabetes . . .

Campers with diabetes need to do a little extra planning. Food and all the necessary (and a little extra) insulin and blood glucose testing supplies should be carefully packed and taken along with you. Don't assume that there will be a food source nearby if you experience low blood glucose. Also, be sure to wear your medical identification.

Because physical activity usually lowers blood glucose levels, canoers, hikers, or backpackers will need to increase their food intake to allow for the increased activity. In general, begin by increasing calories by twenty percent. On days of very strenuous activity, you may need to eat an extra 1000 calories a day. Snacks are always important, but even more so with increased activity. Weariness can decrease appetite at a time when extra food is important. Turn your lunch into small, frequent snacks eaten throughout the day to provide a steady flow of fuel without overloading your stomach. Fruit rolls and low-fat granola bars are handy, healthy sources of carbohydrate to bring along. If you take insulin, your doses may need to be decreased as well. Your health care provider can help you decide how to do this. Reduce only the insulin that's working during the time of your activity.

Sample Camping Menu

Menu	Exchanges
Breakfast	
Cooked cereal, biscuit, toast, pancakes, or french toast	4–5 starch, 3–4 fat
Fruit juice or dried fruit	1–2 fruit
Cocoa	1 other carb
Dried egg powder	1–2 meat
Morning Snack	
Granola	2–3 starch, 2–3 fat
Lunch	
RyKrisp®	2–3 starch
Raisins	2–3 fruit
Hard salami, cheese, or peanut butter	2–3 meat
Artificially sweetened Kool-Aid®	free
Afternoon Snack	
Graham crackers, RyKrisp®, gorp, or granola bar	2–3 starch, 2–3 fat
Dried fruit, raisins	2–3 fruit
Artificially sweetened Kool-Aid®	free
Dinner	
Casserole using meat	4–5 starch, 4–5 meat
Biscuits or dessert	1–2 starch, 1–2 fat
Dried vegetables	veg, as desired
Dried fruit	1–2 fruit
Evening Snack	
Crackers, biscuits, or popcorn	2–3 starch, 1 fat
Cheese, peanuts, or sunflower seeds	1–2 meat
Dried fruit	1–2 fruit
Dried milk or cocoa	1 milk
Daily Total	
Exchanges:	18 starch, 9 fruit, 2 milk, 1–2 veg, 10 meat, 9 fat
Calories:	3400
Carbohydrate:	440 grams (53%)
Protein:	145 grams (17%)
Fat:	115 grams (30%)

CAMPING FOOD LIST

Food	Quantity	Carbohydrate Choices	Exchanges
Starch			
Biscuits	1 biscuit (2")	1	1 starch, 1 fat
Cereal, cooked	½ cup	1	1 starch
Chow mein noodles	½ cup	1	1 starch, 1 fat
Corn	½ cup (1 oz dried)	1	1 starch
Cornbread	2" square	1	1 starch, 1 fat
French toast	1 slice	1	1 starch, ½ med. fat meat
Graham crackers	3 squares	1	1 starch
Hash browns, cooked	½ cup (2 oz dried)	1	1 starch, 2 fat
Hushpuppies	1 ball (2")	1	1 starch, 1 fat
Pancakes			
6" across	1 pancake	1	1 starch, 1 fat
4" across	3 pancakes	1	2 starch, 1 fat
Potatoes			
Mashed	½ cup (3 oz dried)	1	1 starch
Diced	½ cup (2 oz dried)	1	1 starch
Rice, cooked	⅓ cup	1	1 starch
RyKrisp®	3 crackers	1	1 starch
Saltine® crackers	6 crackers	1	1 starch
Soup	1 cup	1	1 starch
Fruit			
Dried fruit	¼ cup (½ oz)	1	1 fruit
Fruit galaxie	¼ cup	1	1 fruit
Juice	½ cup	1	1 fruit
Prunes	3 medium	1	1 fruit
Raisins	2 Tbsp (½ oz)	1	1 fruit
Stewed fruit	½ cup	1	1 fruit
Milk			
Dried nonfat milk powder	⅓ cup powder	1	1 skim milk

Food	Quantity	Carbohydrate Choices	Exchanges
Other Carbohydrates			
Brownie	2 x 4" piece	2	2 other carb, 2 fat
Cake, white or yellow, no icing	3" square	2	2 other carb, 2 fat
Cookies	3" across	1	1 other carb, 1 fat
Fruit bars	1 bar	1½	1½ other carb
Fruit rolls or roll-ups	1 roll (½ oz)	1	1 other carb
Gingerbread	3 x 2" piece	2	2 other carb, 2 fat
Gorp	⅓ cup	1	1 other carb, 1 fat
Granola	¼ cup	1	1 other carb, 1 fat
Granola bar	1 small bar	1	1 other carb, 1 fat
Marshmallows	2 large	1	1 other carb
Pudding	½ cup	2	2 other carb
S'mores	1 s'more	3	3 other carb, 1 fat
Syrup, real maple	¼ cup	4	4 other carb (1 Tbsp = 1 other carb)
Light	2 Tbsp	1	1 other carb
Tang® or other fruit drinks, as prepared	½ cup	1	1 other carb
Vanilla wafers	5 wafers	1	1 other carb
Vegetable			
Vegetables, dried	½ cup (1 oz dried)	0	1 veg
Meat/Meat Substitutes			
Beef jerky	½ oz	0	1 very lean meat
Beef			
Canned	2–3 oz	0	3 lean meat
Dried	2 oz	0	3 med. fat meat
Dried, chipped	2–3 oz	0	3 lean meat
Cheese	1 oz	0	1 high fat meat

Food	Quantity	Carbohydrate Choices	Exchanges
Chicken			
Canned	2–3 oz	0	3 lean meat
Dried	2 oz	0	3 lean meat
Cold cuts	1 slice (1 oz)	0	1 high fat meat
Eggs, prepared	⅓ cup	0	2 med. fat meat
Ham	1 oz	0	1 lean meat
Meat sticks	½ oz	0	1 lean meat
Meat, canned	4 oz	0	3 med. fat meat
Peanut butter	1 Tbsp	0	1 high fat meat
Peanuts	¼ cup (1 oz)	0	1 high fat meat, 1 fat
Pork chops, dried	2 oz	0	2 med. fat meat
Salami	1 slice (¼" thick or 1 oz)	0	1 high fat meat
Sardines, canned	1 oz	0	1 lean meat
Sausage patties	2 oz	0	2 high fat meat
Shrimp, canned	1 oz	0	1 lean meat
Spam®	1 slice (3 oz)	0	3 high fat meat
Sunflower seeds	¼ cup (1 oz)	0	1 high fat meat, 1 fat
Tuna fish, canned in water	½ can (3–4 oz)	0	3 very lean meat
Combination Foods			
Baked beans and franks	1 cup	2	2 starch, 2 high fat meat
Beef stew	1 cup	1	1 starch, 2 med. fat meat, 1–2 fat
Beef stroganoff	1 cup	2	2 starch, 2 med. fat meat, 1–2 fat
Chicken à la king	1 cup	1	1 starch, 2 med. fat meat, 2 fat
Chicken and dumplings	1 cup	2	2 starch, 2 med. fat meat, 1 fat
Chili with beans	1 cup	2	2 starch, 2 lean meat
Chow mein (without noodles or rice)	2 cups	2	2 starch, 1 veg, 2 lean meat

Food	Quantity	Carbohydrate Choices	Exchanges
Lasagna	1 cup	2	2 starch, 2 med. fat meat
Macaroni and cheese	1 cup	2	2 starch, 1 high fat meat
Spaghetti and meatballs	1 cup	2	2 starch, 1 veg, 2 med. fat meat
Tuna noodle casserole with peas	1 cup	2	2 starch, 1 veg, 2 med. fat meat

APPENDICES

Resources

Nutrition

The American Dietetic Association

216 West Jackson Boulevard, Suite 800
Chicago, IL 60606
(312) 899-0040 or (800) 877-1600
www.eatright.org/
This organization also has a diabetes education division
called the Diabetes Care and Education Dietetic Practice
Group.

Diabetes

American Diabetes Association

1660 Duke Street
Alexandria, VA 22314
(800) 232-3472
www.diabetes.org/

Canadian Diabetes Association

15 Toronto Street, Suite 800
Toronto, ON M5C2E3 Canada
(416) 363-3373
www.diabetes.ca/

American Association of Diabetes Educators

444 North Michigan Avenue, Suite 1240
Chicago, IL 60611
(312) 644-2233 or (800) 338-3633
www.aadenet.org/

International Diabetes Center

3800 Park Nicollet Boulevard
Minneapolis, MN 55416-2699
(612) 993-3393
www.idc.org/

Juvenile Diabetes Foundation International

120 Wall Street, 19th floor
New York, NY 10005
(212) 785-9500

National Diabetes Information Clearinghouse

1 Information Way
Bethesda, MD 20892

Heart Disease

The American Heart Association

7272 Greenville Avenue
Dallas, TX 75231
(214) 373-6300 or (800) 242-8721
www.amhrt.org/

National Cholesterol Education Program Information Center

4733 Bethesda Avenue, Suite 530
Bethesda, MD 20814-4820

Camping

Alpine Aire

PO Box 926
Nevada City, CA 95959
This organization makes freeze-dried camp food.

Mountain House

Oregon Freeze Dry Inc.
PO Box 1048
Albany, OR 97321
This organization makes freeze-dried camp food.

Travel

International Association for Medical Assistance to Travelers

417 Center Street
Lewiston, New York 14092
(716) 754-4883
This organization can provide a list of doctors in foreign countries who received postgraduate training in North America or Great Britain. See chapter 9 for more information.

International Diabetes Federation

40 Washington Street
B-1050 Brussels, Belgium
This organization can provide a list of International Diabetes Federation groups that can offer assistance when you're traveling.

APPENDIX 2

More On Fat Replacers

Fat replacers can be grouped according to what they are made from—carbohydrate, protein, or fat—or according to the number of calories they contribute to the diet. Some are calorie-reduced substitutes while others are calorie free. Calorie-reduced substitutes are made by replacing lower-calorie carbohydrates or proteins for fat. They are digested and absorbed normally and provide one to four calories per gram. (Fat provides nine calories per gram.) Because they have long been used in foods for other purposes, the FDA classifies these products "GRAS"—generally regarded as safe—and does not require manufacturers to conduct safety studies on them.

Fat Replacers Made From Carbohydrate

For more than a decade, some carbohydrates have been used to partially or totally replace fats or oils in a wide variety of food products. The carbohydrate-based fat replacements include dextrins, maltodextrins, modified food starches, polydextrose, cellulose, and gums. Dextrins and modified food starches are bland, nonsweet carbohydrates that when water is added form gels that mimic the texture of fat. They can be derived from wheat, potato, corn, tapioca, rice, or combined starches.

Polydextrose is a nonsweet starch made from dextrose and small amounts of sorbitol and citric acid. It was initially developed as a bulking agent for non-nutritive sweeteners but can also replace up to one-half of the fat in a product. Microcrystalline cellulose is made from purified wood pulp processed to form a gel. It can replace a percentage of fat in salad dressings and frozen desserts.

Gums such as xanthane gum, guar gum, carageenans, and water can also be used to stabilize the consistency of foods in place of fat. Algins from kelp are also used as stabilizers in liquid salad dressings. They are not digested so the calories are negligible.

Fat Replacers Made From Protein

Through a process called microparticulation, proteins such as egg white or whey protein can be changed to have characteristics of fat as well. In this process, protein is heated and blended to create very, very small round particles. These particles flow over the tongue to create a rich, creamy taste similar to fat. It supplies one and one-third calories per gram compared to nine calories per gram from fat. It can't be used in products that will be heated, such as oils used for frying or for most baking. Heat causes the protein to gel and lose its creamy consistency.

The NutraSweet Company, manufacturer of aspartame, has developed Simplesse as a fat replacer. It is a microparticulated egg white and milk protein product. Dairy-Lo is another fat replacer made from a whey protein concentrate that can be used in a few baked products. K-Blazer, Lita, and Veri-Lo are other protein-based fat replacers.

Microparticulation does not change the protein in any way uncommon to cooking. The body digests and absorbs these products like any other protein. These products are therefore safe for anyone who does not have sensitivities to egg or milk products.

Fat Replacers Made From Fat

Olestra (Olean) is an example of a calorie-free fat replacement. It is a combination of sugar and oils brought together by a process combining high temperature and pressure. Because the resulting molecule has a larger size and shape, the body's digestive enzymes are unable to break it down, and it cannot be absorbed into the bloodstream and converted to calories. However, it has the same taste and cooking properties as regular oils and fats. Olestra can be used wherever fats are used, even in high temperature cooking such as baking and deep frying. The FDA has approved the use of olestra in snacks.

Caprenin is a fat substitute made from fat that is currently being used in food products. It has properties similar to those of cocoa butter and so is used in candies and in confectionery coatings for nuts, fruits, cookies, and so on. Unlike other fats that supply nine calories per gram, caprenin provides five calories per gram. Salatrim (Benefat) is a new family of low-calorie fats which are only partially digestible and not fully absorbed. Salatrim also contains only five calories per gram. It can replace fat in chocolate and confections, cookies and crackers, dairy products, and snacks.

Other calorie-free fat replacers made from fats have very long names and are usually abbreviated with the use of initials. None of these products has yet been approved by the FDA.

APPENDIX 3

Common Sugars and Sweeteners

Brown sugar. Made by exposing sugar crystals to a molasses syrup with natural flavoring and color or by simply adding syrup to refined white sugar in a mixture. It is ninety-one to ninety-six percent sucrose.

Corn syrup. Produced by the action of enzymes and/or acids on cornstarch. It is the liquid form of corn sugar and, when crystallized, may be called corn syrup solids or corn sweetener.

Dextrin. A sugar formed by the partial breakdown of starch.

Dextrose. Also called corn sugar. It is made from starch by the action of heat and acids or by enzymes. It is often sold for commercial use blended with regular sugar.

Fructose. Also called fruit sugar or levulose. It occurs naturally in small quantities in fruit. It has four calories per gram, as do all carbohydrates. Fructose is sometimes used in Europe as an alternative to sweeteners, such as sucrose, that contain glucose. Crystalline fructose is a commercial sugar that is sweeter than sucrose, although its sweetness actually depends on how it's used in cooking. If used in products that are cold and acidic in nature, it tastes sweeter. If used in products that require heat, such as baking, it is usually not sweeter than sucrose. Although fructose causes a more modest increase in blood glucose levels than other sugars, it is equal in caloric value and so must be counted as part of the total caloric intake.

Fruit juice concentrate. Concentrated fruit juice that is often used to replace sucrose in jams, jellies, and other sugar-free products. It has little, if any, advantage over sucrose. It is not as sweet as sucrose so more is needed to provide equal sweetening power.

Galactose. Simple sugar found in lactose (milk sugar).

Glucose. The basic sugar found in the blood. It either comes from the digestion and absorption of food carbohydrates, from the breakdown of muscle and liver glycogen, or is manufactured in the liver from other sources such as proteins. It is the form of carbohydrate that the body uses for energy.

High fructose corn syrup (HFCS). HFCS is a combination of fructose and dextrose (glucose) and is a derivative of corn. The amounts of fructose vary and many contain forty-two, fifty-five, or ninety percent fructose. Glucose or dextrose comprise most of the balance. HFCS has an effect on blood glucose similar to that of sucrose. Its increased use is due to the growing market for soft drinks in which HFCS is a major ingredient.

Honey. An invert sugar formed by an enzyme from nectar gathered by bees. Its composition and flavor depend on the source of nectar. Fructose, glucose, maltose, and sucrose are among its components.

Hydrogenated starch hydrolysates (HSH). HSH is produced by a series of chemical reactions that begin with cornstarch. This produces a series of products containing mixtures of polyols (sugar alcohols). The sweetness varies from twenty-five to fifty percent of sucrose and is suitable for use in a variety of candies. It is also known as hydrogenated glucose syrup or hydrogenated sugar.

Invert sugar. A sugar formed by splitting sucrose into its component parts: glucose and fructose. This is done by an application of acids or enzymes. It is used only in liquid form and is sweeter than sucrose. Invert sugar helps prolong the freshness of baked foods and confections and is useful in preventing food shrinkage.

Lactose. The sugar found naturally in milk, which is a combination of glucose and galactose. For commercial purposes it is made from whey and skim milk. The pharmaceutical industry is a primary user of prepared lactose.

Maltose. Comes from the breakdown of starch in the malting of barley.

Mannitol. A sugar alcohol manufactured from mannose and galactose. It is half as sweet as sucrose. It is commonly used as a bulking agent in powdered foods and as a dusting agent for chewing gum. Excessive consumption may cause diarrhea.

Maple syrup. A syrup made by concentrating the sap of the sugar maple tree.

Molasses. The thick, brown syrup that is separated from raw sugar in its manufacture.

Polyols. Another name for sugar alcohol; they are synthetic products made from "ose" sugars. Instead of contributing four calories per gram like other sugars they contribute on average two calories per gram.

Raw sugar. Tan to brown in appearance, it is a coarse, granulated solid obtained by evaporating the moisture from sugar cane juice.

Sorbitol. A sugar alcohol made commercially from glucose or dextrose. It is about half as sweet as sucrose and is the most commonly used sugar alcohol. It is readily converted to fructose and is similarly used by the body. One of the major problems with sorbitol is that it may cause diarrhea in some people. Also, many products sweetened with sorbitol contain as many or more calories than the product they are replacing because of the added fat used to dissolve the sorbitol and give the food a creamy texture.

Sorghum. Syrup from the sweet juice of the sorghum grain.

Sucrose. Crystals from cane or beet sugars. It is composed of two simple sugars, glucose and fructose. Sucrose is almost one hundred percent pure and sold either granulated, cubed, or powdered.

Turbinado sugar. Sometimes viewed erroneously as raw sugar. It actually has to go through a refining process to remove impurities and most of the molasses. It is produced by separating raw sugar crystals and washing them with steam.

Xylitol. A sugar alcohol manufactured from xylose (wood sugar from part of the birch tree). Its sweetness is about equal to sucrose.

Calculating Exchanges From Food Labels

The Exchange Lists group foods according to their nutritional content. Each serving of food on a given list contains about the same carbohydrate, protein, fat, and calories. The table below shows the nutrient values for each exchange list.

Nutrient Values of Food Exchanges

Groups/Lists	Carbohydrate (grams)	Protein (grams)	Fat (grams)	Calories
Carbohydrate				
1 starch	15	3	1 or less	80
1 fruit	15	–	–	60
1 milk (skim)	12	8	0–3	90
1 other carbohydrates	15	varies	varies	varies
Vegetable				
1 vegetable	5	2	–	25
Meat and Meat Substitutes				
1 very lean	–	7	0–1	35
1 lean	–	7	3	55
1 medium-fat	–	7	5	75
1 high-fat	–	7	8	100
Fat				
1 fat	–	–	5	45

The following Nutrition Facts information is from a twelve-inch frozen pizza topped with ground beef. To convert this information into exchanges, you need to consider the serving size and the carbohydrate, protein, and fat values. The number of grams in the food do not have to be exactly equal to the numbers shown in the table. In most meal plans, variations of a few calories or grams of carbohydrate, protein, or fat are not significant. Follow the steps below to figure out how to count this food in a meal plan based on exchanges.

Serving Size ⅓ pizza (113 g)
Calories 310
Total Fat 16 g
Total Carb 27 g
Sugars 3 g
Protein 14 g

Step 1. Check the serving size. Is this a reasonable amount for you to eat? Remember that all the Nutrition Facts information is based on this serving size. If you eat double the serving size, you will eat twice as much carbohydrate, protein, fat, and calories.

Step 2. Look at the grams of carbohydrate in the serving size. Ask yourself: What kind of carbohydrate is in the food? In this case, the carbohydrate comes from the pizza crust, so it is a starch. You'll be converting the carbohydrate to starch exchanges. Note in the table on page 283 that one starch exchange equals fifteen grams of carbohydrate and three grams of protein. Because the pizza in this example has twenty seven grams of carbohydrate, you can count all of the carbohydrate as two starches. Each starch exchange also has three grams of protein, so you need to subtract six grams of the protein from the total amount of protein in the serving size.

	Carbohydrate	Protein	Fat
	27 g	14 g	16 g
2 starch exchanges =	30 g	- 6 g	− 0 g
		8 g	16 g

Step 3. Now you have eight grams of protein and sixteen grams of fat left. The table shows that meat exchanges contain protein and fat. This pizza is topped with ground beef, which is on the Medium-Fat Meat List. One medium fat meat exchange has seven grams of protein and five grams of fat. Subtract these amounts from the remaining protein and fat.

	Carbohydrate	Protein	Fat
	27 g	14 g	16 g
2 starch exchanges =	30 g	− 6 g	− 0 g
		8 g	16 g
1 medium-fat meat exchange =		7 g	− 5 g
			11 g

Step 4. The remaining eleven grams of fat will count as fat exchanges. Each fat exchange has five grams of fat.

	Carbohydrate	Protein	Fat
	27 g	14 g	16 g
2 starch exchanges =	30 g	- 6 g	0 g
		8 g	16 g
1 medium-fat meat exchange =		7 g	- 5 g
			11 g
2 fat exchanges =			10 g

If you choose to eat one-third of this pizza, you would count it as two starches (two carbohydrate choices), one medium-fat meat, and two fats in your meal plan.

Foreign Language Phrases for People With Diabetes

French

I am a diabetic.	Je suis diabétique.
I am on a special diet.	Je suis au régime spécial.
I need some sugar.	J'ai besoin de sucre.
Without sugar	Sans sucre
Sugar added	Avec le sucre
I take daily injections of insulin.	Je prends chaque jour une piqûre d'insuline.
Please get me a doctor.	Allez chercher un médecin, s'il vous plâit.
Sugar or orange juice, please.	Sucre ou jus d'orange, s'il vous plâit.

German

I am a diabetic.	Ich bin Zuckerkrank. Ich bin Diabetiker (M), Diabetikerin (F).
I am on a special diet.	Ich halte eine Sonderdiät ein.
I need some sugar.	Ich brauche etwas Zucker.
With sugar	Mit Zucker
Without sugar	Ohne Zucker
Sugar added	Zucker hereingestellt
Low calorie	Kalorienarm
No calories	Ohne Kalorien
Low fat	Fettarm
I take daily injections.	Täglich nehme ich Insulinspritzen of insulin.

Please get me a doctor.   Rufen Sie mir bitte einen Arzt.
Sugar or orange juice, please.   Zucker oder Orangensaft, bitte.

Italian
I am a diabetic.   Io sono diabetico.
Please get me a doctor.   Per favore chiama un dottore.
Sugar or orange juice, please.   Succhero o succo d'arrangio, per favore.

I take daily injections of insulin.   Predo injectiones de insulin tutti giorni.

Norwegian
I am a diabetic.   Jeg har sukkersyke.
I am on a special diet.   Jeg har en spesielle diet.
I need some sugar.   Jeg trenger sukker.
With sugar   Med sukker
Without sugar   Utenfor sukker
I take daily injections of insulin.   Jeg tar sproytene daglig.

Spanish
I am a diabetic.   Yo soy diabético (M), diabética (F).

I am on a special diet.   Estoy a dieta especial.
I need some sugar.   Neccesito azúcar.
Without sugar   Sin azúcar
Sugar added   Con azúcar
Low calorie   Poca calória
No calories   Sin calórias
Low fat   Poca grasa
I take daily injections of insulin.   Tomo inyecciones diarias de insulina.

Please get me a doctor.   Hágame el favor de llamar al médico.

Sugar or a glass of orange juice, please.   Azúcar o un vaso de jugo de naranja, por favor.

APPENDIX 6

Glossary of Food Terms

Abalone:
A delicate, bland-tasting mollusk often used in main dishes.

Achar:
Indian brine-pickled fruits and vegetables, e.g., limes, lemons, mangoes, green beans, and green chiles.

Ackee:
Although the ackee is a fruit, it is usually cooked and served as a vegetable. When cooked its taste is similar to scrambled eggs.

Adzuki beans:
A small brownish bean used frequently in Japanese cooking and often served mixed with brown rice or other grains.

Agemono:
Japanese word meaning "deep-fried things."

Alfredo:
An Italian creamy cheese sauce.

Almond butter:
A spreadable paste made from ground, toasted almonds.

Alu mattar:
Indian curried potatoes and peas.

Alu paratha:
Flat whole wheat Indian bread with spiced potato filling.

Amaranth:
A grain originally used by the ancient Aztecs, now often used combined with other grains. The seeds are yellowish brown and tiny (each kernel is about the size of a poppy seed). It can be used as a thickener for soups and stews.

Antipasto:
Spicy Italian meats, seafoods, and/or vegetables arranged on a platter and served cold as an appetizer.

Appam:
Deep-fried Indian pancake made of rice, lentils, and flour.

Apple banana:
Also called manzano or finger bananas. They are finger sized and turn black when ripe.

Arroz con pollo:
Rice with chicken, tomatoes, and spices.

Arroz:
Spanish word for rice.

Artichoke:
Globe artichokes are large, unopened buds from a thistle-like plant. You eat them by pulling off the leaves one by one from the cooked artichoke and drawing them between your teeth. The tender heart can be eaten whole. The fuzzy choke at the center should be cut or scooped out and discarded.

Asafetida:
A strong-smelling sap or resin from the roots of various East Indian plants. Powdered, it is used in very small amounts in lentil dishes and meat stews.

289

Ashgourd:	Pumpkinlike vegetable with light green skin and white flesh.
Atole:	A hot Mexican beverage made of milk or water, sugar, and cornstarch thickener. Vanilla, cinnamon, chocolate, or other flavors may be added.
Bagel:	A hard yeast roll shaped like a doughnut.
Balsamic vinegar:	Vinegar made from the juice of white grapes. Its dark color and sweet/sour flavor come from aging for several years in wooden barrels.
Balushahi:	Crisp, sweet Indian pastry fried in ghee, then dipped in sugar syrup.
Barfi:	An Indian sweet with a fudgelike texture made from milk and sugar and flavored with vanilla or cardamom.
Barley:	Pearl barley refers to the refined product with the bran removed and the kernel steamed and polished. Both regular and quick barley are available. Mild in flavor and use in soups, main dishes, and salads.
Bean sprouts:	Tiny white bean shoots with pale green hoods that come from the soya, mung, or curd bean. They may be eaten raw or cooked.
Besan:	Chickpea flour.
Bhindi:	Indian word for okra.
Bhuna:	An Indian dish consisting of chicken, beef, or lamb roasted with spices, onions, and tomatoes.
Bialy:	A Jewish breakfast roll that is flat and softer than a bagel.
Biryani:	An Indian dish consisting of shrimp, lamb, or vegetable layered with basmati rice and vegetables.
Bitter melon (balsam pear):	Cucumber-like vegetable with a bumpy green surface and bitter flavor.
Black beans, fermented:	A tangy spice used in Chinese cooking to darken sauces or as a main ingredient.
Black mushrooms:	Dried fungi used extensively in Chinese cooking. Also known as Chinese or winter mushrooms.
Blintzes:	A Jewish dish consisting of very thin, rolled crepe usually filled with cottage cheese, pot cheese, or a fruit mixture.
Bok choy:	Vegetable with broad white or greenish-white stalks and loose, dark-green leaves. Also known as Chinese chard or white mustard cabbage. It resembles both Swiss chard and celery.
Bolillo:	Similar to a French roll. May replace tortillas or be used to make a sandwich.
Bolognese:	Named after the town of Bologna, Italy, it refers to dishes served with a thick, full-bodied meat and tomato-based sauce. Wine or cream are sometimes added.
Borscht:	Soup made with beets, cabbage, or other vegetables and sour cream. It may be served hot or cold.

Bottle gourd:	Pale green, large bulb-shaped, thick skinned vegetable with thick pulp.
Breadfruit:	Starchy and melon-shaped, it is used as a vegetable in Caribbean and Latin American cooking. It is boiled or baked like a potato and has a taste similar to bread, which is how it gets its name.
Brewer's yeast:	A savory, powdered flavoring used as a supplement in cooking. It does not rise like regular yeast.
Bruschetta:	Pizza or bread dough seasoned with herbs and baked. Served with Italian meals in wedges with toppings such as chopped tomatoes and garlic.
Bubke:	Jewish coffeecake that is yeast-risen and sweetened with cinnamon and sugar.
Buckwheat:	A bushlike plant. Buckwheat seeds are called groats, coarse ground groats are called grits, and finely ground groats are buckwheat flour.
Bulgur:	Whole wheat kernels that have been steamed, dried, and crushed. They cook very quickly and have a chewy texture and slightly nutty flavor. Use in pilaf and other side dishes and soups.
Bulke:	A Jewish yeast roll that is large, light, and softer than a bagel.
Burrito:	A soft flour tortilla filled with beans, ground beef, chicken, or cheese. It is rolled and covered with a sauce or deep-fried.
Cactus fruit:	Also known as a prickly pear fruit.
Cactus leaves:	*see* Nopales
Café con leche:	Spanish phrase for coffee with milk.
Calabacitas:	Mexican squash that is similar in size and shape to the cucumber and has light-green skin. Often simmered with onion and spices and/or combined with meat in a casserole dish.
Cannelloni:	An Italian dish consisting of hollow pasta filled with ricotta cheese, meat, and/or spinach and served with cheese and tomato sauce.
Canola oil:	Comes from rapeseed, a member of the mustard family. The name is an abbreviation for "Canada oil" because its oil seed was developed in Canada. Extremely clear and light and is often used in formulated foods because of its bland flavor.
Caper:	The unopened flower bud on a bush native to the Mediterranean region. Gathered and sun-dried, they are preserved by pickling in a vinegar brine or packed in salt, which gives them a pungent flavor.
Carambola (star fruit):	Glossy, yellow pods marked with five longitudinal ribs that form a star shape when the fruit is sliced crosswise. It has a golden yellow color with juicy flesh and crisp texture.

Carbonara:
An Italian bacon, egg, and cheese sauce served with pasta.

Cardamom:
Spice made from the dried fruit of a plant of the ginger family. The pods or seeds are used in meat, rice, and some dessert dishes. One of the most expensive but common spices used in curries.

Carne guisada:
Beef tips sautéed with chopped onions, green pepper, and chili peppers. Stewed tomatoes are added and the combination is simmered until tender.

Carne:
Spanish word for meat.

Carob:
A long, edible sweet pod that grows on an evergreen tree in the Mediterranean region. The pod can be ground and used in baked products. It is often used as a chocolate substitute because it tastes like cocoa. It is also called carob bean, honey bread, or locust bean.

Cassava:
Large, starchy root with a bitter odor that disappears after cooking. The starch derived from this root is used to make tapioca. Also called manioc or Yucca root.

Cellophane noodles:
Hard, opaque, fine, white noodles made from ground mung beans.

Ceviche:
A Mexican dish of marinated seafood.

Challah (hallah):
A loaf of very light Jewish egg bread, often braided and usually prepared for the Sabbath and holidays.

Chana dahl:
Dahl made from chickpeas.

Chapati or puppodum:
A thin, grilled, pancake-shaped whole wheat bread, popular in Indian cookery, made with or without fat.

Chayote:
Mexican squash that is light green, pear-shaped, and sometimes covered with tiny hairs. It can be used in any recipe that calls for winter or summer squash.

Cheese foods:
At least fifty-one percent of the product is pasteurized processed cheese, with cream, milk, skim milk, or whey added.

Cheese spreads:
These are cheese foods with an edible stabilizer and extra moisture added to allow smooth spreading at room temperature.

Chestnuts:
A nut that has a hard, brown outer shell and an inner shell that protects the kernel. To shell, make a deep x on the flat side; cover with boiling water, and simmer two to three minutes; drain two to three nuts at a time; and pull off shells and inner skins. To roast, make a deep x on flat side; roast in a fireplace, place nuts on edge of open fire or in a long-handled popcorn basket. Shake over fire until they pop.

Chicken cacciatore:
An Italian dish consisting of sautéed chicken pieces simmered in a meatless tomato sauce.

Chicken tikka:
An Indian dish consisting of bite-size pieces of chicken cooked in clay ovens with charcoal.

Chile rellenos:	A Mexican dish of green chile peppers filled with cheese and wrapped in a rich egg batter. Deep-fried and smothered in chili verde.
Chiles:	Refers to the chile pepper, of which there are over 100 varieties ranging in flavor from mild to sweet to pungent to red hot. Used fresh, canned, or dried, or as an ingredient in sauces or dishes.
Chili con carne:	Commonly referred to as chili. A hearty soup made with tomato, onions, peppers, kidney beans, spices, and beef.
Chili paste:	Condiment made with mashed chile peppers, vinegar, and garlic.
Chili powder:	Blend of chiles, herbs, and spices.
Chimichanga:	A Mexican dish consisting of a flour tortilla filled and folded like a burrito, then deep-fried.
Chinese cabbage (Nappa):	A member of the cabbage family, it has a long slender head with long, pale green and white wrinkled leaves. It has a tender texture and a mild, delicate flavor.
Chirimoya:	A heart-shaped fruit with a rough, green outer skin. When ripened and chilled, the flesh has a sherbetlike texture. Also called sweet sop, sherbet fruit, or custard apple.
Chole:	Indian word for chickpeas. Aloo chole is chickpeas cooked with tomatoes and potatoes.
Cholent:	A slow-cooking Jewish stew that can be prepared with or without meat.
Chorizo:	A highly seasoned sausage of chopped beef or pork with sweet red peppers. Frequently fried and eaten in a taco, burrito, or tortilla mixed with scrambled eggs.
Chow chow:	Small bulblike vegetable with rough, light-green skin and white pulp used in Indian cooking.
Chow luny aas:	A Chinese dish which is lobster tails in garlic sauce.
Chutney:	Highly seasoned relish or accompaniment made from raw, cooked, or pickled fruits or vegetables and/or coconut.
Cilantro:	The fresh leaves and stems of the coriander plant.
Cioppino:	An elaborate Italian fish stew.
Coconut milk:	A creamy liquid extracted by grating fresh coconut meat (not the liquid inside the coconut).
Colocasia:	Lotuslike plant that grows in water or marshy places. Cooked and used as a vegetable in India.
Congee:	A Chinese soupy rice gruel which is usually served with side dishes such as pickled vegetables, salted eggs, and fish. Other ingredients such as meat, fish, and vegetables can be added. A sweet version may also be prepared by adding sugar and lotus seeds.

Coriander:	Spice with a pungent, musky flavor. Its fresh, leafy version is known as cilantro or Chinese parsley.
Corn oil:	Comes from the germ—or innermost part—of the corn kernel. It has a slightly sweet taste.
Cottonseed oil:	Nation's top-selling oil until 1930s. Today it is not readily available in stores.
Couscous:	Tiny cream-colored granules of finely milled wheat with a soft texture and buttery flavor. It can be cooked quickly by a soak and steam method and is a nice substitute for rice.
Curry:	A mixture of individually roasted spices used in Indian cooking.
Dahi (curds):	Unflavored yogurt eaten at most Indian meals as an accompaniment, either plain or mixed with vegetables.
Dahl (dal), raw:	Raw dahl is a pulse (edible seed) resembling the common split pea used in India. Dahl also refers to a light, spicy puree made of many kinds of dried beans, peas or lentils; for example, chana dahl is made from chickpeas; mung dahl is made from mung beans.
Daikon:	A large white radish that can be served raw or pickled. The flavor is slightly hotter than an ordinary radish.
Dim sum:	Chinese steamed or fried dumplings stuffed with meat, seafood, and/or vegetables, sweet paste, or preserves and often served at brunch.
Donburi:	A Japanese dish served on a bed of rice with special sauce.
Dosa:	Indian pancake-like bread made from fermented rice flour and lentils and sometimes stuffed with vegetables.
Drumstick:	Narrow, long, fibrous, green Indian vegetable used in curries.
Duck eggs, preserved:	Chinese duck eggs soaked in brine for thirty to forty days.
Duck feet:	A Chinese dish of duck feet braised in soy sauce, sugar, wine, salt, monosodium glutamate, and spices.
Duck sauce:	A Chinese sauce made by blending plums, apricots, vinegar, and sugar. Also known as plum sauce.
Egg roll:	Minced or shredded meat and/or seafood and vegetables wrapped in egg roll wrapper and deep-fried.
Eggplant:	A dark purple, glossy, and pear-shaped vegetable which originated in the Orient.
Enchilada:	A Mexican dish consisting of an oil-blanched corn tortilla folded (or rolled) around a filling of beef or cheese. It can be covered with a sauce of chili con carne, tomato, cheese, or guacamole and garnished with chopped onions and grated cheese.

Enchirito:	A Mexican dish consisting of an enchilada with meat, chiles, beans, and sauce.
Ensalada de aquacite:	A Mexican salad of sliced avocado with tomato and lettuce.
Fajitas:	A Mexican dish consisting of chicken, beef, or shrimp sautéed with onions, peppers, tomatoes, and Mexican spices. Served in a skillet, with flour tortillas and salsa on the side.
Falafel:	Patties made from coarse-ground wheat germ, garbanzo beans, fava beans, and spices, then lightly fried in oil.
Farfel:	Noodle dough grated into barley-sized grains and served in soup.
Feijoa:	It looks like an elongated guava and has an aromatic pulp that combines the taste of pineapple, quince, spruce, and Concord grapes with a menthol-lemon tang. The inside is eaten fresh or used as an ingredient in fruit salads and jams.
Fennel:	Another spice used in curries, also referred to as sweet cumin. Commonly used in sweet dishes or tea.
Fettuccine Alfredo:	Thin, flat pasta served with a creamy cheese sauce.
Fidelio con carne:	A Mexican dish consisting of sautéed beef cubes combined with browned vermicelli, tomatoes, and spices.
Filled Milk:	Milk that contains fats or oils other than milk fat.
Firni:	A sweet Indian pudding made of milk, cream of rice, and nuts.
Fish maw:	A Chinese dish wich is dried and deep-fried stomach lining of fish.
Fish sauce:	A Chinese sauce made by fermenting small, salted fish in wooden casks for several months and draining the liquid.
Flan (Mexican custard):	A sweetened egg custard topped with caramelized sugar.
Flanken:	Flank steak.
Flauta:	A rolled, filled, fried corn tortilla.
Fleishig:	Yiddish word for meat and meat products. Also used to describe meals that include meat.
Florentine:	A dish garnished with or containing finely ground spinach.
Foccacia:	Italian flat, round bread sometimes flavored with herbs.
Frijoles:	Spanish word for beans. Served in some form at nearly every meal in Mexico, they are frequently simmered until tender with onion, cilantro, chile pepper, diced tomatoes, and seasonings.
Frijoles cocidos:	Boiled beans.

Frijoles refritos:	Refried beans. Prepared by simmering beans with bacon, onion, garlic, whole tomatoes, cilantro, and herbs until soft, then mashing and frying them slowly. Chili powder may be added.
Frittatta:	Italian omelet topped with sautéed vegetables and/or sausage.
Fung gawn aar:	A Chinese dish which is made up of shrimp, chicken liver, and mushrooms in chicken broth.
Fusilli primavera:	An Italian dish of spiral, long pasta topped with sautéed vegetables.
Garam masala:	A blend of dried ground spices, usually black peppers, cumin, coriander, cloves, ginger, cinnamon and others used in Indian cooking.
Gazpacho:	A pureed vegetable soup usually served cold.
Gefilte fish:	A highly seasoned chopped freshwater fish such as carp, pike, or whitefish mixture that is blended with eggs and matzo meal.
Ghee:	Butter that has been clarified or gently warmed over low heat until it browns lightly, giving it a distinct aroma. It is used as a flavoring or as a topping for rice and breads.
Ginkgo nuts or seeds:	Small fruit of Ginkgo tree with tough, beige-colored shells and ivory-colored nuts used in Asian dishes.
Glutinous rice:	Popular in Japan and other Asian countries, it is a short-grained, pearl white rice that becomes sticky and translucent when cooked. Also known as sweet or sticky rice.
Gnocchi:	An Italian dish of little dumplings made from white flour, potato, or a combination of both, and often topped with sauce.
Granadilla (passion fruit):	It has the size and shape of an egg, a tough purple skin, and yellow flesh with black seeds and appears shriveled when ripe and ready to eat. It reminded early South American missionaries of Christ's crown of thorns, so they named it passion fruit.
Grebenes:	Rendered chicken fat and chicken skin fried with onions.
Greens (cooking):	Mild flavored greens include beet tops, dandelion, spinach, and collards. Strong-flavored greens include kale, mustard, Swiss chard, and turnip tops.
Guacamole:	Mashed avocado mixture sometimes seasoned with salsa, chopped chiles, and other seasonings.
Guava:	A sweet, juicy fruit whose skin ranges in color from green to yellow with an inside that can be white, deep pink, or salmon red. It has many small seeds in the center and is native to Mexico and South America.
Halva:	A very sweet Indian dessert made from milk, vegetables such as carrots or pumpkin, and sometimes nuts.

Hamantaschen (purim tart):	Three-cornered Jewish cakes made with pastry or cookie crust and filled with poppy seeds, dried fruit, or cheese.
Hang mung poo:	Spicy steamed mussels.
Harina:	Spanish word for flour.
Hoisin sauce:	Also known as Chinese barbecue sauce, it is a sauce made from fermented mashed soybeans, salt, sugar, and garlic.
Homli fruit:	A cross between a grapefruit and an orange. It has a greenish skin with orange flesh. The fruit is slightly sweeter than a grapefruit but not as sweet as an orange.
Huevos reales:	A Mexican dessert made with egg yolks, sugar, sherry, cinnamon, pine nuts, and raisins.
Hummus:	A spread made from pureed garbanzo beans (chickpeas), tahini, lemon juice, olive oil, and garlic.
Idli:	A flattened, cupcake-shaped Indian bread made from ground lentils and rice, and steamed in small saucers.
Italian green beans:	Wide, quick-cooking green beans often served in a sauce.
Jerusalem artichoke:	North American native tuber from the sunflower plant. It has a sweet, nutty flavor and can be served raw or boiled and used as a potato substitute.
Jícama:	A large, lumpy tuber with dull brown skin and a crisp, white, juicy flesh. It has a flavor similar to water chestnuts and is delicious when eaten raw.
Kalamato olives:	Black Greek olives slit so the wine-vinegar mixture in which they are soaked will penetrate.
Kasha:	Buckwheat groats served as a cooked cereal or as a potato substitute.
Kashrut:	The Kosher dietary laws based on the Torah.
Katsuo:	A basic ingredient of Japanese stock, it is made from dried bonita (fish belonging to the mackerel family).
Kayaku goban:	Japanese dish consisting of vegetables and rice.
Kefir:	A cultured dairy product similar to milk.
Kheema do pyaza:	An Indian dish consisting of curried ground lamb or beef with onions.
Kheema mattar:	An Indian dish consisting of curried ground lamb or beef and peas cooked in a spicy sauce.
Khir (kheer):	A sweet Indian pudding made of milk and long-grain rice and flavored with cardamom.
Kichlach:	Light egg cookies.
Kishke:	Yiddish word for beef casings stuffed with seasoned filling that is made from matzo, flour, fat, and onions.

Kiwifruit: Brown and elongated with a fuzzy skin, the inside is lime green and similar in texture to the American gooseberry. It is also known as a "Chinese gooseberry" because of its Chinese origin. It now comes from New Zealand or California.

Knaidlach: Matzo balls made of matzo meal, eggs, and fat, usually served in chicken soup.

Knish: Yiddish word for pastry (sometimes potato-based) filled with ground meat, potato, or kasha and spices.

Kofta: An Indian dish consisting of vegetables, cheese, and ground meat such as lamb that is shaped like a meatball, fried, and curried.

Kohlrabi: A member of the cabbage family with a delicate, turnip-like taste. Bulbs may be steamed or eaten raw.

Korma: A curried Indian dish with a thickened nut-and-yogurt sauce.

Kreplach: Bite-sized Jewish pastry filled with meat or cheese mixture, similar to ravioli.

Kuchen: German word for coffeecake; popular in Jewish cooking.

Kugel: Pudding or casserole, commonly made with potatoes or noodles in Jewish cooking.

Kulcha: Leavened baked Indian bread.

Kumquat: A tiny, oval-shaped, yellow-orange fruit of Chinese origin. It has a very definite citrus flavor. The skin is sweet and the flesh has a tangy flavor. The seeds should be removed before eating.

Lactaid: Lactose, which is milk sugar, is reduced, usually to three grams per cup. Often useful for people with a lactose intolerance.

Lasagna: An Italian dish consisting of very wide, flat pasta layered with meat, cheese, and tomato sauce.

Latkes: Yiddish word for pancakes. Potato latkes are very popular.

Lauki: An Indian bottle gourd.

Lecithin: Extracted from soybeans and used as a dietary supplement.

Leckach: Jewish honey cake.

Leeks: They resemble green onions in shape and flavor but are much larger and milder.

Legumes: Dried beans (kidney, garbanzo, navy, pinto, lima), peanuts, black-eyed peas, and lentils.

Lobia: Indian word for black-eyed peas.

Lokshen: Yiddish word for noodles.

Longan: A small, round Asian fruit with a smooth, brown skin and clear pulp. Fresh longans come in clusters, but the canned product is more common.

Loquat: A small, round fruit with yellow-orange skin and pale yellow to orange flesh with black seeds. Although it resembles an apricot, it has a flavor like a blend of banana and pineapple. It comes from a tropical, ornamental evergreen tree, is very juicy, not too sweet, and is best eaten ripe.

Lotus root: Tuberous stem of the water lily used in Asian dishes such as salads, stir fries, or cooked in soups or stews.

Lox: Smoked, salted salmon that is cut very thin.

Lychee (lichee, litchi): An ancient Chinese fruit that is small, delicate, juicy, and round. It has a reddish brown, hard skin that is easy to peel. The flesh is white and mild flavored with a single seed and has the consistency of a fresh grape. It is used as dessert, as a garnish, or in sweet and sour dishes.

Macadamia nut: Nut from the tall evergreen silk-oak tree; hard-shelled, shiny round nut with delicate flavor. Grown in Hawaii.

Macaroni: Short noodle. Two ounces dried measures one half cup and yields one and one third cups cooked measure.

Machli aur tamatar: Indian curried halibut.

Maize: Spanish word for corn.

Malai: A thick cream that is made from milk by separating and collecting the top part of boiled milk. Used in Indian entrées for a thick, creamy sauce.

Malanga: Large herb with a starchy, thick, tuberous, white, edible root.

Mango: Mangoes may vary in size and shape, depending on the variety and area in which they are grown. They are generally large and oval-shaped with a tough skin that can be green, yellow, red, or a combination of the three, with more reds and yellows as the fruit ripens. Their flesh is orange-yellow, has a spicy aroma, and a rich flavor that is a blend of apricot and pineapple. They must be fully ripe before eating.

Manicotti: Large, tubular pasta filled with meat or cheese and served with meatless tomato sauce.

Manteca: Spanish word for lard.

Marinara sauce: A meatless Italian tomato sauce made with garlic, onions, and oregano.

Marsala: A sweet dessert wine often used in preparations or desserts.

Masa harina: Specially-prepared corn flour used to make corn tortillas, tamales, and nachos.

Masala: An Indian dish consisting of chicken, beef, lamb, fish, or shrimp cooked in a thick spicy yogurt and curry sauce.

Masala dosa: A crepelike Indian pancake with spiced potato filling.

Mattar paneer: An Indian dish of green peas with cottage cheese.

Matzo: Flat, unleavened cracker.

Matzo farfel:	Barley-sized matzo grains.
Matzo meal:	Finely ground matzo used in cooking and baking.
Meat analogs:	Foods made of vegetable protein that duplicate the flavor, texture, and appearance of meat.
Melons:	*Cantaloupe (muskmelon):* A melon with a cream-colored netting over golden undercolor, orange flesh color, and a distinctive-sweet flavor, musky-sweet aroma.
	Casaba: Large round melon with deeply furrowed, yellow rind and a creamy white flesh. Tastes similar to honeydew, has little aroma.
	Golden honeydew: Golden tinge to its skin, orange-like colored flesh, juicy and similar to a cantaloupe.
	Honeydew: Waxy skin, white and green outside, inside has a cream to pale green flesh and a juicy, sweet, honey aroma.
	Orange honeydew: Shaped like a honeydew, it has a soft orange color to its skin with a salmon-colored flesh.
	Pink honeydew: Pink tinge to its skin, pinkish flesh, juicy. Tastes sweet and has a honey-like aroma.
Menudo:	A tripe and hominy soup that is a popular weekend breakfast dish in Mexico.
Mexican rice:	White rice sautéed in a skillet with tomatoes, green peppers, onions, and seasonings.
Milchig:	Yiddish word for milk or dairy foods. Also used to describe meals that include dairy products.
Millet:	A tiny, round, yellowish grain widely used in Asia and Africa. Often served as a simple grain dish tossed with chopped onions and herbs.
Minestrone:	A thick vegetable and pasta soup.
Miso:	A fermented soybean paste with a salty, earthy flavor that is made by combining soybeans, and sometimes a grain such as rice, salt, and a mold culture and then aged. The addition of different ingredients and variations in length of aging produce different types of miso that vary in flavor, texture, color and aroma. Miso can be used to flavor soups, sauces, dressings, and marinades, and to make pâtes.
Mock duck:	A Chinese vegetarian mixed dish that commonly consists of wheat gluten cooked with vegetables.
Mole:	A Mexican sauce or gravy of dried red chiles, chocolate, chicken broth, cinnamon, sesame seeds, nuts, and other spices. Served on special occasions, this sauce is usually cooked with chicken or turkey and served with tortillas, beans, and rice.
Mum yee mein:	A Chinese dish consisting of braised noodles, chicken breast, mushrooms, chestnuts, and Chinese peas.

Naan (nan): Individual leavened flat Indian bread made of white flour, and traditionally baked in a clay oven.

Nachos: Fried tortilla chips with cheese.

Natto: Fermented, cooked soybean with a sticky, viscous coating and a cheesy texture.

Natural cheeses: Curds (milk solids) are pressed into "natural" cheese. They may or may not be aged or ripened to make different types of cheese. The milk liquid (whey) is either discarded or recycled to make mysost, primost, ricotta, or other whey-based cheeses. It may also be used for cottage cheese or cream cheese.

Nopales (cactus): The leaves or pods of the prickly pear cactus, which are sliced in strips and cooked with onions and spices. They taste like crisp green beans. To prepare, remove the "eyes" which contain cactus thorns with a sharp knife; cut leaves into cubes and cook in water for ten minutes.

Nori: A sea vegetable sold in flat, dried sheets for Japanese dishes. Often used to make sushi or nori rolls.

Oats: A member of the grass family. The inedible hulls are removed, leaving the groats.

Oat bran: An oat cereal product especially milled to concentrate the protein, vitamins, and minerals found naturally in whole grain oats.

Old-fashioned rolled oats: Made from oat groats that are steam-cooked, then flattened.

Quick-cooking rolled oats: Made by steam-cooking, cutting, and flattening groats.

Steel-cut oats: Oat groats that have only been cut, rather than rolled out. Very crunchy.

Okra: Slim, tapered pods that are sometimes nicknamed "lady's fingers." Okra can be used as a thickening agent in soups or stews.

Olive oil: Most of the world's olive oil is produced in the Mediterranean region.

Extra virgin: The highest grade, it must come from top-quality grapes. The fruit is hand-harvested, washed, blended, and mashed. The mash is squeezed at room temperature in a hydraulic press—"cold pressed." Oil is separated from the watery part and graded by acidity and by taste. It can be called Extra Virgin only if it meets certain standards for color, aroma, and flavor, and passes a chemical test: It must contain less than one percent free oleic acid, a fatty acid that can damage olive oil's flavor. If the acidity is a little higher the oil can be designated Virgin or Superfine Virgin.

Light or extra light: Olive oil that is simply refined oil without much of an olive flavor.

Pure: Oil that can't pass for virgin and oil from less carefully culled fruit, it still has a distinct olive flavor.

Orzo:	Rice-shaped pasta. Two ounces dried measures or.e half cup and yields one cup of cooked orzo.
Oyako:	Sautéed chicken, eggs, and onions.
Pakora:	An Indian dish consisting of deep fried, spicy vegetable (cauliflower, eggplant, potato, lentils, etc.) or chicken fritter.
Pan dulce:	Mexican sweet bread or sweet rolls served at breakfast or as an afternoon or evening snack. Generally lower in fat and sugar than the American equivalent.
Paneer:	Homemade Indian cottage cheese used in curries, vegetable and rice dishes, and desserts. Made from milk that is curdled with lemon juice and then strained through cheese cloth.
Papaya:	It is really a very large berry with a deep green outer peel and yellow-to-orange inside. It has a mild flavor and contains an enzyme, papain, that is extracted and sold as a tenderizer. It can be eaten fresh or cooked.
Paratha:	Unleavened bread made from wheat flour and cooked on a grill. It may be spread with oil or butter during or after cooking. Parathas can also be stuffed with vegetables such as potatoes, cauliflower, radish, spinach, or dahl.
Pareve:	Yiddish word for neutral foods such as fish, eggs, fruits, and vegetables, which may be served at either a meat or a dairy meal.
Parmigiana:	A granular textured parmesan cheese that is aged two years.
Pasta:	Fresh or dried flour-based noodles available in a variety of shapes, including fettuccine, linguine, spaghetti, cannelloni, macaroni, elbow, shells, rigatoni, rotelle, vermicelli, etc. Two ounces of dried pasta—regardless of shape—is a reasonable portion for most adults.
Peanut oil:	Produced largely from nut fragments not suitable for other purposes such as peanut butter. It has a mild to nutty flavor.
Pear, Asian:	Originally from China, it looks like a very small pear. Crisp and russeted, it is also known as apple-pear, Japanese pear, pear-apples, and Chalea.
Persimmon:	A bright orange fruit with a shiny skin that is removed before eating. Known as the "apple of the Orient." Persimmons must be very soft before eating or they have a very sour, astringent taste.
Pescado:	Spanish word for fish.
Pesce:	Italian seafood.
Pesto:	A basil, cheese, and nut paste usually served with pasta.
Phoa:	Indian rice that has been pounded into ragged, translucent flakes. Eaten with milk as a cold cereal, or plain or deep-fried as a snack.

Phulka:	Round, puffed, whole-wheat Indian bread, made without fat and cooked directly over a very low gas flame.
Picadillo:	A type of beef that is flavored with traditional Spanish ingredients of olives and raisins, as well as Caribbean tomatoes and hot chiles.
Picante:	The Mexican word for "hot and spicy."
Pine nut:	Edible sweet flavored nut produced in the pine cone of the nut-bearing pine tree; looks like a large grain of rice. Also called pinon or pignolia.
Pirogi or piroshkes:	Pastry filled with cheese or meat.
Pistachio nut:	Seed of a red fruit that has a double shell. The natural color of the seed is green.
Plantain:	A greenish banana with a rough, blemished skin which remains starchy even when fully ripe. It is an important staple food in tropical countries. Used as a vegetable, the fruit is starchy and is never eaten raw. It can be baked, boiled, or prepared in much the same way as potatoes.
Po tak:	A Japanese dish of hot and sour seafood in lemon juice.
Poi:	A thick paste with a starchy, mild taste made from the ground, cooked roots of the taro plant.
Polenta:	An Italian dish which is a cornmeal and water mixture, baked and served with a sauce.
Pomegranate:	The name means "apple with many seeds." It is about the size of an orange with a hard skin and deep red color. The inside is filled with edible sweet seeds which are the only edible part of the fruit; the pulp is too bitter.
Pomelo:	This citrus fruit, the tropical ancestor of the grapefruit, has a thick rind and sweet, red pulp. The flavor is mild rather than bitter.
Pot cheese:	Cream cheese or other farmer-style cheese.
Prickly pears:	The fruit of a species of cactus; also called cactus pear, Indian fig, and Barberry fig. It has a yellow to crimson skin that is covered with spines. The inside is purple-red to yellow and has a sweet taste similar to watermelon.
Primavera:	Italian sautéed vegetables.
Processed cheeses:	American, cheese food or cheese spreads are a blend of one or more natural cheeses that are ground, blended, or heated together. This process provides uniformity of product and increases the shelf life.
Prosciutto:	An Italian ham that has been salt-cured, seasoned and air-dried (not smoked). It is pressed to produce a firm texture and is sliced very thin.

Pullaos:	Indian dishes: plain pullao is basmati rice cooked with saffron; peas pullao is basmati rice cooked with peas and spices; shrimp pullao is basmati rice cooked with shrimp and spices.
Pulse:	The edible seeds of various leguminous crops such as peas, beans, or lentils.
Puppodums (papadam):	Very light, puffed, crisp Indian wafers made from spicy lentils and served as a side dish or appetizer.
Puri:	Thin, deep-fried, whole-wheat Indian bread.
Quesadillas:	Tortillas filled with cheese and heated or fried until cheese melts. They are eaten with salsa, usually as snacks.
Queso fresco, blanco, or mexicano:	White, crumbly, Mexican cheese that is low in fat. Similar to cottage cheese.
Quince:	A very ancient fruit that has hard, tart meat that is not good for eating. Quince is best when made into a sauce or baked.
Quinoa:	A tiny, millet-like seed used as a grain, originally from South America. It has a soft texture and sweet, nutty flavor. Before cooking, always rinse the grain well to remove a slightly bitter coating. Serve as a hot cereal or side dish, use in salads, baked goods, or add to soups.
Raita:	A saladlike combination of yogurt with grated cucumbers (or other raw or cooked vegetables), onions, and spices that is eaten in India.
Rajmah:	Indian curried, cooked red beans.
Ramaki:	Chicken livers and water chestnuts wrapped in bacon.
Ras malai:	An Indian dish of paneer (cheese) balls boiled in condensed milk and sugar.
Ratatouille:	Tomatoes, eggplant, and zucchini cooked in olive oil.
Ravioli:	An Italian dish consisting of pasta squares stuffed with eggs, vegetables, cheese, or meat and covered with tomato sauce.
Rice:	In converted white rice, the unhulled grain is steamed, resulting in some of the nutrients being pushed into the grain. Some starch is also removed. Different sizes differ in texture when cooked.
	Arborio rice: An Italian short-grain rice that when cooked has the ability to absorb large amounts of liquid and still retain a firm texture.
	Basmati rice: An aromatic long grain rice, native to India and Pakistan. Slightly nutty flavor.
	Brown rice: The entire grain with only the outer husk removed. Slightly nutty flavor and chewy texture. Requires a longer cooking time than white long grain rice.
	Texmati rice: A domestic Basmati rice grown in the United States.

	Wild rice: Not really a rice, but an aquatic grain-like seed from a North American grass. Nutty flavor. Varies in color from dark brown to dark black. Versatile for use in breads, salads, soups, main and accompaniment dishes and desserts.
Rice noodles:	Very thin strands of translucent noodles often sold in coiled nests. When deep fried they become crunchy and airy. They are often used in oriental salads or they can be presoaked and used in soups and stir-fries.
Rice vermicelli:	Thin, white noodles made from rice flour, often used as an alternative to rice.
Risotto:	Italian short-grain rice that has a creamy consistency when cooked; often mixed with butter and cheese before serving.
Roti:	Indian breads, including chapati, dosa, idli, kulcha, naan, paratha, phulka, and puri (see individual definitions).
Rugalah (strudel):	Thin pastry rolled up in fruit and nut filling.
Saag paneer:	An Indian dish of spinach cooked with cottage cheese.
Sablefish:	Though it is commonly called "black cod," this northern Pacific fish is not cod. A high fat content gives it a soft texture and a rich taste that is surprisingly mild.
Safflower oil:	Comes from perhaps the world's oldest crop, a thistle grown for centuries in India. It is used to make premium margarines.
Saffron:	Spice obtained by drying the threadlike, deep-orange stamens of the saffron crocus. Known as the most expensive spice in the world, saffron is used in small quantities in Indian cooking.
Salsa:	A combination of tomato, chiles, and onions. Depending upon the chilies used, flavor ranges from mild to fiery hot.
Salsify:	Also known as vegetable oyster or oyster plant. It is a grassy, flat, green plant with pale tan flesh and an oyster flavor.
Sambhar:	An Indian dish consisting of lentil puree cooked with vegetables and spices.
Samosa:	Deep-fried Indian pastry filled with a mixture of vegetables or meat.
Sapodilla:	A fruit with a rough, brown skin and sweet slightly grainy flesh. Eaten when fully ripe.
Sapota:	Also called the Mexican custard apple, sapotas resemble green apples in appearance. Clusters of the fruit are large and greenish-yellow. It has a custard-like consistency and flavor that some believe tastes like vanilla ice cream, and it can be eaten fresh.
Sashimi:	A Japanese dish of sliced raw fish.
Schav:	Jewish soup made from sorrel that is similar to borscht.

Schmaltz:	Rendered chicken fat, often used in cooking or pastry making.
Sesame oil:	Untoasted oil is yellow, toasted is brown. It has a taste that ranges from bland to powerfully sesame-like, depending on the variety. Oil made from toasted seeds is very pungent.
Shabu shabu:	A Japanese dish of sliced beef and vegetables that is cooked and served at the table with noodles and a special sauce.
Shami kebab:	Indian fried patty made of ground meat.
Shiu mi:	A Chinese dish of chopped chestnuts, chives, and pork wrapped in thin noodles.
Shrikhand:	An Indian sweet made of curds, sugar, and flavoring such as cardamom.
Shrimp scampi:	Large shrimp seasoned with oil.
Shumai:	Japanese steamed dumplings.
Snow peas:	These are sometimes called sugar peas or Chinese peas and have transparent green pods.
Soba noodles:	Japanese noodles made from buckwheat.
Sofrito:	A combination of onions, garlic, cilantro, sweet chiles, and annato seeds. It serves as a base for many Mexican dishes as well as an all-purpose sauce.
Sopa:	A Mexican side dish consisting of rice, pasta, and sometimes tomatoes cooked in consommé. It also can be a dessert when Mexican sweet bread is added.
Sorrel:	A member of the buckwheat family. Cooked as a green, leafy vegetable.
Soybean:	A high-protein, high-fat bean used to make a variety of products such as tofu, tempeh, tamari, miso, soymilk, and textured vegetable protein.
Soybean oil:	Light in flavor with almost no odor, it is the natural oil extracted from whole soybeans. It is the most frequently consumed oil in the United States. It is used in eight-three percent of all margarines and sixty-two percent of all salad dressings, and it represents eighty percent of all salad and cooking oils.
Soymeat:	Spun soy protein products. The cheeselike curd from soybeans is mechanically manipulated to obtain a meatlike texture.
Soymilk:	The rich creamy milk of whole soybeans has a unique nutty flavor and can be used in a variety of ways. It is available as a plain, unflavored beverage or in a variety of flavors including chocolate, vanilla, carob, and almond.

Spaetzle:
: A German side dish served in place of potatoes or rice and often accompanied by a sauce or gravy. It is made from flour, eggs, and water or milk, formed into tiny noodles or dumplings by either rolling the dough or forcing it through a sieve, and then usually boiled.

Spaghetti:
: Long noodle. Two ounces of dried long noodles yields one cup cooked spaghetti. Two ounces of dried pasta held in a fist would make a circle exactly the size of a U.S. penny.

Spanish rice:
: White rice sautéed in a skillet with tomatoes, green peppers, onions, and seasonings.

Spanish sauce:
: Diced peppers, either mild or hot, are soaked, seeded, and ground to a paste. Herbs, spices, vegetables, and meat or poultry stock are added to make a fairly heavy paste or puree.

Spring roll wrapper:
: Thin sheets made from rice flour; larger than wonton wrappers and often used for Vietnamese egg rolls.

Spumoni:
: Chocolate and vanilla ice cream with a layer of rum-flavored whipped cream containing nuts and fruit.

Squash, summer:
: They have soft shells and include:

: *Pattypans (scallop or button):* They are disc-shaped with a ribbed edge, giving them a scalloped appearance. The skin is pale green when young, white when older. The entire squash can be eaten.

: *Spaghetti:* An edible gourd that is light green in color with a smooth skin.

: *Straightneck:* They are similar to the crookneck but relatively straight.

: *Yellow crookneck:* They have a warted, light yellow skin with a creamy yellow flesh and are curved at the neck.

: *Zucchini (Italian squash):* Straight in shape with a skin color that is dark green.

Squash, winter:
: They have hard, firm shells and are higher in calories than summer squash. A one-cup cooked portion is included on the starch list. Winter squash include:

: *Acorn:* It is acorn-shaped with yellowish, sweet tasting flesh. It is usually cooked unpeeled because of its tough skin.

: *Banana:* It is cylindrical in shape and has a pale olive gray color that changes to creamy pink in storage. It is usually sold by the piece.

: *Buttercup:* Drum-shaped with a turban cap at the blossom end, it has green skin and bright yellow-orange flesh.

: *Butternut:* Cylindrical in shape with a bulbous base, it has dark yellow skin and yellow orange flesh.

: *Hubbard:* Heavy for its size, it has a bright yellow-orange flesh and is usually sold by the piece.

Mediterranean: A long cylindrical shape and slightly bulbous at one end, it is beige in color with a ridged skin and bright orange interior. Also sold by the piece.

Succotash:
A dish of North American Indian origin consisting of corn and beans.

Suimono soup:
A clear, broth-type Japanese soup.

Sukiyaki:
A Japanese meat and vegetable dinner.

Sunflower oil:
Though the sunflower is native to the American Southwest, Russia leads the world in sunflower production. It is good for every use; its oil flavor does not overpower foods.

Sushi:
A Japanese dish consisting of rice mixed with rice vinegar, often served with sliced raw fish (sashimi).

Szechwan:
A style of Chinese cooking characterized by use of fiery pepper sauces.

Tabouli:
A Middle Eastern salad made from bulgur and flavored with lemon and mint.

Taco:
A crisp, deep-fried corn tortilla folded in half to hold seasoned ground beef, diced tomatoes, shredded lettuce, and cheese.

Tahini:
Sesame seed paste.

Tamales:
Extruded, cooked corn flour wrapped around a chili beef filling. A sauce of chili con carne, tomato, or cheese can be used as an accompaniment.

Tamari:
Soy sauce made in the traditional Asian way, which requires long periods of fermentation and aging.

Tamarind:
Fruit with a long, flattened, cinnamon-brown pod. Usually used dried or as pulp in cooking to impart a sweet-sour taste.

Tamata salat:
An Indian dish of diced tomatoes and onions with hot spices and lemon.

Tandoori chicken:
An Indian dish consisting of chicken roasted in clay ovens with charcoal. Tandoori chicken has a red color on top from the spices and cooking.

Tandoori:
Cylindrical clay ovens heated with charcoal used in Indian cooking.

Tangelo:
A citrus fruit with loose skin that is a hybrid of the tangerine. It is the size of a large orange, but the flavor is slightly more tart.

Taro root:
Starchy, tuberous, rough-textured brown root. Also known as dasheen, tannia, eddo, malanga, and tannier. Commonly used in Hawaii and eaten in the form of poi. Cooked taro ranges in color from purple to cream.

Teiglach:
A Jewish dish consisting of small balls of sweet dough cooked in honey.

Tempeh:
Whole soybeans, usually mixed with another grain such as rice, millet, or barley, that are fermented and pressed into a solid cake. It has a dense, chewy texture. It is found in the frozen food case and can be marinated and grilled, barbecued, or baked in sauces. Also used in soups, casseroles, and salads.

Tempura:
A Japanese dish consisting of deep-fried fish, shellfish, or vegetables.

Teriyaki:
A Japanese method of cooking using a sweet soy-seasoned glaze.

Textured vegetable protein (TVP):
A name for textured soy protein, which is made from soy flour. Available in granules or chunks, this product is sometimes flavored to taste like meat and is used in place of ground beef in recipes.

Tofu:
Soft, unripened cheeselike curd made from soybeans. It can be stir-fried, steamed, grilled, baked, or scrambled, or used in dressings, dips, desserts and pasta sauces.

Tomatillos:
Commonly known as ground tomatoes, they are small, firm, round, husk-covered green vegetables. When eaten raw they have a tart taste.

Tonkatsu:
Japanese fried pork.

Tortilla:
The bread of Mexico. Baked, flat, round, thin cakes of unleavened cornmeal (masa) or wheat flour.

Tostadas:
Tortillas that have been fried until golden brown and crisp in hot lard or oil. They are served with various combinations of meat, poultry, sauces, chiles, lettuce, and tomatoes.

Traif (trefe):
Jewish foods that are non-kosher, forbidden, and ritually unfit.

Tropical oils:
Two kinds of palm trees—coconut palm and the oil palm—provide most of the world's supply of palm-derived oils. Coconut oil comes from the nut of the coconut palm and palm oil and palm kernel oil are produced from the fruit and nuts, respectively, of oil palm tree. These oils are about ninety percent saturated fatty acids.

Turmeric:
A spice from the ginger family that gives the yellow-orange color to commercial curry.

Tzimmes:
Versatile Jewish hot side dish often made with dried fruit, carrots, and sweet potatoes, and sweetened with honey. Tzimmes may be prepared with meat and served as a main dish or made with fruit and served as a dessert.

Udon noodles:
Flat whole wheat noodles used in Asian cooking.

Ugli fruit:
Native to Jamaica, it is about the size of a grapefruit with a disfigured, rough peel. The skin peels off like a tangerine and the pulp is very juicy with an orange-like flavor.

Upma:
An Indian breakfast item made with cream of wheat or fuji spices, and sometimes with vegetables.

Veal cacciatore:	An Italian dish consisting of veal cutlet topped with tomato sauce and sautéed onions, mushrooms and peppers.
Veal parmigiana:	An Italian dish consisting of thin slices of veal, pounded for tenderness, rolled in bread crumbs and Parmesan cheese, and covered with mozzarella cheese and a meatless tomato sauce.
Veal piccata:	Medallions of veal lightly sautéed in a butter, lemon, and wine sauce.
Verdolaga (purslane):	A Mexican vegetable with tender leaves and young stalks that can be eaten in a salad or cooked like spinach.
Vindaloo:	An Indian dish consisting of chicken, beef, lamb, or fish cooked with potatoes and hot spices.
Water chestnuts:	They are brown on the outside and have a white inside with a nutlike flavor. They remain crisp even after cooking and are commonly used in Chinese cooking.
White clam sauce:	Italian white-wine-based cream sauce containing whole clams.
Wonton:	A steamed or fried wrapper filled with minced pork and/or shrimp.
Wonton wrappers:	Thin, yellow sheets made of flour, egg, salt, and water used in Chinese cooking.
Yaki-udon soup:	A Japanese buckwheat noodle soup with stir-fried vegetables.
Yakitori:	A Japanese dish which is chicken teriyaki.
Yard-long beans:	Thin, flexible, tender beans that can grow to a length of up to eighteen inches. Related to black-eyed peas in appearance, taste, and texture, they are perfect in long-cooked dishes and add a chewy, firm, almost meaty texture and taste.
Yautia:	A starchy, edible tuber that is cooked and eaten like yams or potatoes.
Yu hsiang chicken:	A Chinese dish consisting of strips of chicken stir-fried with bamboo shoots, water chestnuts, wood ears, lily buds, and Chinese cabbage.
Zita:	Medium-short noodle. Two ounces dried measures one cup and yields one and one-half cup cooked zita.
Zuppe:	Italian soup.
Zuppa de pesce:	Italian fish soup.

References

Ahuja, S. R. 1991. *Diabetic Bhog.* 2d ed. New Delhi, India: B.I. Publications Pvt. Ltd.

American Institute for Cancer Research. 1992. A la grecque, a la king, a la what? A guide to restaurant terms. *American Institute for Cancer Research Newsletter* (Winter).

Cooper, N. 1991. *The joy of snacks.* Minneapolis: Chronimed Publishing.

Franz, M. J. 1990. Alcohol and diabetes. Parts 1 and 2. *Diabetes Spectrum* 3:136-144, 2210-215.

———. 1991. Nutrition: the cornerstone. In *Learning to live well with diabetes,* ed. M. J. Franz, D. D. Etzwiler, J. O. Joynes, and P. A. Hollander, 21-48. Minneapolis: Chronimed Publishing.

———. 1997. *Fast food facts.* 5th ed. Minneapolis: IDC Publishing.

Franz M. J., and N. Cooper. 1991. Meal planning: Adding flexibility. In *Learning to live well with diabetes,* ed. M. J. Franz, D. D. Etzwiler, J. O. Joynes, and P. A. Hollander, 305-320. Minneapolis: Chronimed Publishing.

Franz, M. J., B.K. Hedding, and G. Leitch. 1985. *Opening the door to good nutrition.* Minneapolis: Chronimed Publishing.

Gadia, M. 1997. *Lite and luscious cuisine of India.* Ames, Iowa: Piquant Publishing.

Grigson, J., ed. 1984. *The world atlas of food.* New York: Exeter Books.

Human Nutrition Information Service of the United States Department of Agriculture. 1976-1990. *Composition of foods.* Agriculture Handbook Series, no. 8:1-22. Washington, D.C.: United States Department of Agriculture.

Kahn, A. P. 1989. Keeping kosher. *Diabetes Self-Management* (March/April): 33-41.

Kittler, P.G., and P. Sucher. 1989. *Food and culture in America.* New York: Van Nostrand-Reinhold.

Margen, S., and the Editors of the University of California at Berkeley *Wellness Letter.* 1992. *The wellness encyclopedia of food and nutrition.* New York: Random House.

Messina, M., and V. Messina. 1996. *The dietitian's guide to vegetarian diets, issues and applications.* Gaithersburg, Maryland: Aspen Publishers.

Monk, A., and N. Cooper. 1997. *Convenience food facts: A quick guide for choosing healthy brand-name foods in every aisle of the supermarket.* Minneapolis: IDC Publishing.

Pearson, J. 1991. Planes, trains, and automobiles: plan your way to a fun-filled vacation. *Living Well with Diabetes* (Summer): 15–16.

Pennington, J. A. T. 1994. *Bowes and Church's food values of portions commonly used.* 16th ed. Philadelphia: J.B. Lippincott.

Roth, H. 1990. *Guide to low-cholesterol dining out.* New York: Penguin Books.

Sane, T., V.A. Koivisto, P. Nikkanen, and R. Pelkonen. 1990. Adjusting of insulin doses of diabetic patients during long distance flights. *Br Med J* 301:421-422.

The American Dietetic Association and American Diabetes Association. 1989-1996. *Ethnic and Regional Food Practices* (series): *Chinese American, Jewish, Mexican American, Indian & Pakistani.* Chicago: The American Dietetic Association.

Warshaw, H. S. 1990. *The restaurant companion: A guide to healthier eating out.* Chicago: Surrey Books.

Index

A

Accepted daily intake (ADI), sugar substitutes, 44
Acesulfame-K, 43, 68
Air travel, food exchanges during, 90–92
Alba milk powders, 122
Alcohol
  composition of beverages, 84–85
  diabetes and, 86–87
Alitame, 44
Amaranth, 167, 172, 192, 197, 289
Amino acids, 164
Anchiote, 150
Arby's fast food exchanges, 234
Asian food exchanges, 175–188
  convenience foods, 244–247
Aspartame, 43, 68

B

Bacon
  fat exchange list, 148–150
  free food exchange list, 151
  meat and meat substitutes exchange list, 137
  simulated bacon, 172
  substitutes, 71
Baking ingredients, 73–76
Barbecue sauce, 151
Beans
  Asian food list, 180, 184–188
  dip, free food list, 151
  exchange list, 101
  fast food exchanges, 234
  Indian food exchanges, 212–218
  Jewish food list, 222
  meat and meat substitutes exchange list, 137
  Mexican-style food exchanges, 192
  vegetarian food list, 168–169, 172
Beef
  meat and meat substitutes exchange list, 137–138

Mexican-style food exchanges, 193–197
Beer, 84
Beverages. *See also* Alcohol; Juices
  alcoholic beverage composition, 84–85
  international travel and, 92
  other carbohydrates exchange list, 126–130
  snack food list, 251–252
  soft drinks, 44, 130
Blood glucose control
  diabetes and carbohydrate counting, 22–23
  meal planning and, 20–21
Boston Market food exchanges, 234
Breads. *See also* Grains
  convenience food exchanges, 246
  starch exchange list, 101–105, 108–109
  Indian food exchanges, 212–218
  Jewish food list, 222
  lactovegetarian menu, 165
  other carbohydrates list, 126–127
  vegetarian food list, 167
Brewer's yeast, 151, 172
Buckwheat, 172
Burger King food exchanges, 235
Burritos, 156
Butter
  as baking/cooking ingredient, 72
  fat exchange list, 150
  Indian food exchanges, 214
  substitutes, 71
Butter Buds, 151
Buttermilk, 122

C

Cake
  convenience food exchanges, 247
  other carbohydrates exchange list, 126–130
  snack food list, 258

Calories
  fat as percentage of, 32–34
  food labels, 56
  meal planning and, 17, 19–21
  in Nutrition Facts Information, 54–55
Camping
  food exchanges, 261–267
  information sources, 272
Candies
  free foods exchange list, 151
  other carbohydrates exchange list, 126–130
Caprenin, 276
Carbohydrates. *See also* Starch; Sugar
  calculating exchanges from, 283
  camping food exchanges, 265
  diabetes and counting of, 22–23
  exchange lists, 97–130
  as fat replacers, 39, 275
  fruit and vegetable lists, 113–120
  function and sources of, 18
  Italian food exchanges, 204–205
  meal planning with, 15–16, 20–23
  Mexican-style food exchanges, 193
  milk exchange list, 121–123
  nutrition facts and counting equations, 59–62
  other carbohydrates exchange list, 125–130
  starch exchange list, 99–111
Carbonated waters
  free foods list, 151–152
  other carbohydrates list, 130
Carob powder, 172
Casseroles, combination foods exchange list, 155–156
Catsup, 152
Caviar, 139
Cereals
  exchange guidelines, 73
  starch exchange list, 102–104

lactovegetarian menu, 165
serving sizes, 100
snack food list, 256
Chapati, 104, 212, 215
Cheese. *See also* Cream cheese
   as baking/cooking ingredient, 72
   camping food exchanges, 265
   Indian food exchanges, 213–214
   meat and meat substitutes exchange list, 139–140
   as milk product, 122
   snack food list, 258
   substitutes, 71
Chewing gum, 152
Chicken
   combination foods list, 156
   fast food exchanges, 230, 234–241, 236–241
   meat and meat substitutes exchange list, 140–141
   Mexican-style food exchanges, 193–197
Chili
   camping food exchanges, 266
   combination foods exchange list, 155–156
   convenience food exchanges, 245–247
   fast food exchanges, 232
   Mexican-style food exchanges, 195–197
Chili sauce, 152
Chimichangas, 156
Chinese foods
   combination foods exchange list, 156
   exchanges and sample menus, 175–176, 178, 180–188
Chips/pretzels/popcorn food exchanges, 252–253
Chocolate and cocoa
   as cooking ingredient, 74–75
   milk list, 122
   other carbohydrates list, 127
   snack food list, 251–252
   substitutes, 71

Cholesterol. *See also* HDL and LDL cholesterol
   fat and, 31–32
   fiber intake and, 49
   meal planning and, 20–21
   saturated fats and, 34–35
   weight loss and, 27
Coconut products, 177, 183, 186–188
Coffee, 151–152
Cold cuts, 140–141
Combination foods
   Asian food list, 183–185
   camping food exchanges, 266–267
   Indian food exchanges, 214
   Italian food exchanges, 205–206
   Jewish food list, 224
   Mexican-style food exchanges, 194–197
Combination foods exchange list, 155–159
Complete proteins, vegetarian exchanges, 164
Condiments, 75, 151–154
   Asian food list, 183, 186–188
   Indian food exchanges, 213–218
   Jewish food list, 223–224
Constipation, 49
Convenience food exchanges, 242–247
Cookies, 126–130, 247
   snack food list, 254–255
Cooking guidelines
   food exchanges and, 67–76
   international travel and, 92
   restaurant food preparation, 78–79
Cooking ingredients, 73–76
Corn food sources, 104. *See also* Tortillas and tortilla chips
Cottage cheese
   lactovegetarian menu, 165
   meat and meat substitutes list, 139
   snack food list, 258
Crackers
   starch exchange list, 104–105
   Jewish food list, 222
   snack food list, 255–256
Cranberries, 152

Cream
   as cooking/baking ingredient, 72
   substitutes for, 71
Cream cheese, 71, 150, 152
Cyclamates, 44

D

Daily servings charts, 19–22
Dairy products. *See* Cheese; Ice cream; Milk and milk products
Dairy Queen food exchanges, 235–236
Desserts. *See also* specific kinds of desserts
   convenience food exchanges, 247
   fast food exchanges, 235, 239–241
   other carbohydrates exchange list, 125–130
Dextrose/dextrin, 279
Diabetes
   alcohol and, 86–88
   camping food exchanges, 262
   carbohydrate counting and, 22–23
   dining out and, 79–80
   foreign language phrases for people with, 287–288
   information sources, 271–273
   meal planning and, 20–21
   sugar consumption and, 42
   travel guidelines, 92–96
   weight loss and, 27
Dim Sum, 184
Dining out
   alcohol and, 84–85
   food choices list, 82–83
   food exchange guidelines, 77–88
   restaurant menu terms, 80–81
Dips, 150, 152
Domino's Pizza food exchanges, 236
Doughnuts, 128

E

Eating habits
   health and, 9–10
   meal planning and, 10–11

Eggs
  Asian food list, 186–188
  as baking/cooking ingredient, 72
  camping food exchanges, 266
  egg salad, 156–157
  exchange guidelines, 74
  meat and meat substitutes exchange list, 142
  substitutes, 71
Enchiladas, 156, 195
Evaporated milk, 71, 122
Exchange lists
  carbohydrates, 97–130
  combination foods, 155–159
  fat list, 147–150
  free food list, 151–154
  fruit and vegetable lists, 113–120
  meal planning with, 11–12
  meat and meat products, 133–146
  milk exchange list, 121–123
  other carbohydrates exchange list, 125–130
  starch exchange list, 99–111
  vegetarian exchanges, 163–173

F

Falafel
  meat and meat substitutes exchange list, 142
  vegetarian food lists, 172
Fast food exchanges, 229–241
Fat replacers, 37–40, 275–277
Fats
  Asian food list, 183
  as baking/cooking ingredient, 72–73
  calculating exchanges from, 283
  cholesterol and, 31–32
  consumption guidelines, 32–34
  diet guidelines for reducing, 36–37
  dining out with exchanges, 79
  exchange guidelines, 74–75
  exchange list, 147–150
  fat replacers from, 37–40, 276–277
  food labeling and, 56–59
  food sources of, 34–35

function and sources of, 18
guidelines for eliminating, 31–40
Indian food exchanges, 214
Italian food exchanges, 205
Jewish food list, 223
meal planning and, 17
meat and meat substitutes exchanges, 133–135
Mexican-style food exchanges, 194
milk exchange list, 121–123
substitutes, 71–72
vegetarian food list, 172
weight control and, 25
weight loss and, 28
Fatty acids, 34–35
Fiber
  guidelines for, 47–50
  sources of, 16
Fish. *See also* Seafood
  Asian food list, 182, 184–188
  combination foods exchange list, 156, 159
  fast food exchanges, 236–241
  Italian food exchanges, 204–206
  Jewish food list, 223
  meat and meat substitutes exchange list, 139, 141–146
  substitutes, 72
Food exchanges. *See also* Exchange lists
  Asian exchanges, 175–188
  camping, 261–267
  convenience foods, 242–247
  cooking with, 67–76
  dining out with, 77–88
  fast food lists, 229–241
  Indian exchanges, 209–218
  Italian exchanges, 201–208
  Jewish food exchanges, 219–226
  meal planning and, 11–12
  Mexican-style exchanges, 189–200
  modifications and substitutions, 68–76
  recipe calculation techniques, 68–76
  snack exchanges, 249–259
  travel and, 89–96
Food Guide Pyramid, 13–14

Food labels
  calculating exchanges from, 283–285
  calories information, 56
  carbohydrate counting, 59–62
  fat information, 56–59
  15-Gram carbohydrate counting equation, 59–62
  guidelines for using, 53–65
  health claims and terminology, 62–64
  ingredients list, 64–65
  nutrition facts, 59–62
  Nutrition Facts Panel, 53–55
  serving sizes, 54–55
Food terms glossary, 289–310
Foreign language phrases, 287–288
Free foods
  Asian food list, 183
  exchange list, 151–154
  Jewish food list, 223
  Mexican-style food exchanges, 194
  vegetarian food list, 172
French toast, 156, 246
Frozen desserts, 128–130
  fast food exchanges, 236–237, 239–241
  Italian food exchanges, 204
  snack food list, 257
Frozen entrees
  combination foods exchange list, 156
  convenience food exchanges, 244–247
Fructose, 279
Fruits
  Asian food list, 181, 186–188
  camping food exchanges, 264
  as cooking ingredient, 75
  exchange list, 114–118
  Indian food exchanges, 213
  lactovegetarian menu, 165
  Mexican-style food exchanges, 193
  snack food list, 256
  substitutes, 71
  sugars from, 279
Fruit spreads
  free foods list, 152–153
  fruit exchange list, 115
  other carbohydrates exchange list, 129

G

Galactose, 279
Gelatin, 72, 129, 152
Glucose
  sources of, 280
  traveling with, 95
Goat milk, 122, 168
Grains
  free foods list, 151
  Jewish food list, 222
  lactovegetarian menu, 165
  starch exchange list,
    105–106, 110–111
  vegetarian food list,
    167–168, 172–173
15-Gram carbohydrate counting equation, 59–62
Gums, 275

H

Ham, 143
Hamburger Helper main
  dishes, 156
Hardee's food exchanges,
  236–237
HDL cholesterol, 31–32
Health claims, on food labels,
  62–64
High fructose corn syrup
  (HFCS), 280
Honey, 280
Horseradish, 152
Humalog insulin, 94
Hummus, 167, 172
Hydrogenated starch
  hydrolysates (HSH), 280
Hydrogenation, fatty acids
  and, 35
Hypoglycemia, 95

I

Ice cream, 129. *See also*
  Frozen desserts, 257
Identification tags and cards,
  87
Illness, travel and, 95
Indian food exchanges,
  209–218
Ingredients
  common baking and cook-
    ing ingredients, 73–76
  list on food labels, 64–65
  modifications and substitu-
    tions, 71–72
  modifying recipes with,
    67–68

Insoluble fiber, 47
Instant Breakfast products,
  129
Insulin, 92–93
Insulin-dependent diabetes
  mellitus (IDDM), 22–23
International Association for
  Medical Assistance to Trav-
  elers (IAMAT), 95–96, 273
Invert sugar, 280
Italian food exchanges,
  201–208

J

Jams and jellies, 152
Japanese food exchanges and
  sample menus, 176–178,
  180–188
Juices
  free foods list, 153
  fruit exchange list, 114–118
  lactovegetarian menu, 165
  other carbohydrates list,
    129–130
  snack food list, 251–252
  sugars from, 279
  vegetable exchange list,
    119–120
  vegetarian food list, 168

K

Kasha, 106, 172
Kefir, 122, 172
KFC food exchanges, 237
Kosher food, 219–226

L

Lactaid, 122
Lacto-ovovegetarians, 163
Lactose, 280
Lactovegetarians
  defined, 163
  sample menu, 165
La Loma vegetarian products,
  169
Lamb, 143
Lasagna, 156
LDL cholesterol, 31–32
Lecithin, 172
Legumes. *See* Beans; Peas
Lentils
  Indian food exchanges,
    212–218
  Jewish food list, 222, 224
  meat and meat substitutes
    exchange list, 143

Lipoproteins, 31–32
Long John Silver's food
  exchanges, 237

M

Macaroni and cheese, 157,
  235, 245
Maltose, 280
Mannitol, 280
Margarine, 149, 153, 165
Matzo products, 222
Mayonnaise
  fat exchange list, 149
  food labeling and, 58–59
  free foods exchange list, 153
  substitutes, 72
McDonald's food exchanges,
  238–239
Meal planning
  alcohol as part of, 87
  calories and, 17, 19
  camping food exchanges,
    262–263
  carbohydrate foods, 15–16
  Chinese food, 176
  convenience food
    exchanges, 242–247
  diabetes and, 22–23
  diabetes and carbohydrate
    counting, 22–23
  dining out and, 77–80
  fast food exchanges,
    229–233
  fat foods, 17
  fat reduction with, 36–37
  guidelines for, 15–24
  Indian food exchanges,
    210–211
  Italian food exchanges,
    201–203
  Japanese food, 176–177
  Jewish food exchanges,
    219–221
  long-term success with,
    23–24
  Mexican-style food
    exchanges, 190–191
  overview of, 10–11
  protein foods, 17
  sample plans, 21
  snack guidelines, 249–251
  travel and, 89–96
  vegetarian exchanges,
    163–164

Meat and meat substitutes
Asian food list, 182–185
calculating exchanges from, 283
camping food exchanges, 265–266
combination foods exchange list, 156–159
as cooking ingredient, 76
exchange list, 133–146
fast food exchanges, 230, 234–241
Indian food exchanges, 213–214
Italian food exchanges, 204–206
Jewish food list, 223
Mexican-style food exchanges, 193
as protein source, 17
snack food list, 258
vegetarian food list, 168–169, 172–173
Menu terms, 80–81
Mexican foods
combination foods exchange list, 156
convenience food exchanges, 244–247
exchange list, 189–200
fast food exchanges, 232, 240–241
Microparticulation, 276
Milk and milk products. *See also* Cheese; Ice cream; Sour cream
Asian food list, 181
as baking/cooking ingredient, 72
camping food exchanges, 264
as common ingredients, 74
exchange list, 121–123
Indian food exchanges, 213
lactovegetarian menu, 165
substitutes, 71–72
sugar from, 279
vegetarian food list, 168
Miso, 106, 143, 173, 187
Monounsaturated fats
fat exchange list, 147–150
food sources, 34–35
meal planning and, 17
Morningstar Farms products, 169

N

Natto, 169, 173
Natural Touch products, 169
Nondairy creamers
fat exchange list, 150
free foods list, 152
Jewish food list, 223
Noodles. *See* Pasta and noodles
Nut butters. *See also* Peanut butter
fat exchange list, 148
meat and meat substitutes list, 144
vegetarian exchanges, 172
Nutrition
carbohydrate counting and, 59–62
elements of, 12–14
information sources, 271
Nutrition Facts Panel, 53–55, 284
Nuts
as cooking ingredient, 76
fat exchange list, 148–150
meat and meat substitutes exchange list, 144
meat and meat substitutes exchanges, 134–135
vegetarian food list, 170

O

Olestra, 37–40, 276–277
Omega-3 fatty acids, 34–35

P

Pancakes, 106, 247
Pasta and noodles
Asian food list, 180–181, 184–188
camping food exchanges, 267
combination foods exchange list, 155–157, 159
as common ingredient, 73
convenience food exchanges, 245–247
exchange list, 106–107
Italian food exchanges, 204–206
Jewish food list, 222, 224
serving sizes and exchanges, 100

Peanut butter
as baking/cooking ingredient, 76
camping food exchanges, 266
fat exchange list, 149–150
meat and meat substitutes list, 144
snack food list, 258
Peas
Indian food list, 212–218
Jewish food list, 222
meat and meat substitutes exchange list, 144
vegetarian food list, 170
Phenylketonuria (PKU), 43
Physical activity
travel and, 94
weight loss and, 28–29
Pie, 130
Pizza
combination foods exchange list, 155, 157
convenience food exchanges, 244–247
fast food exchanges, 231, 236–241
Italian food exchanges, 206
Pizza Hut food exchanges, 239
Polydextrose, 275
Polyols, 281
Polyunsaturated fats
exchange list, 147–150
food sources, 34–35
meal planning and, 17
Pork
Asian food list, 182, 184–185
meat and meat substitutes exchange list, 144–145
Potato chips, 57–58, 108, 252–253
Potatoes
on starch exchange list, 107–108
combination foods exchange list, 155, 157
convenience food exchanges, 244–247
fast food exchanges, 231, 234–241
Jewish food list, 222
Pot pies, 157
Pretzels, 108, 252–253

Protein. *See also* Complete
proteins
    as fat replacer, 39, 276
    function and sources of, 18
    meal planning and, 17
    vegetarian exchanges,
    163–164
Puddings, 126, 130, 259
Puppodums, 108, 212, 217

Q

Quiches, 157
Quinoa, 108

R

Ravioli, 157
Recipes
    exchange calculations for,
    68–70
    healthy modifications to,
    67–68
    modifications and substitu-
    tions, 71–72
Red Lobster food exchanges,
240
Rice
    Asian food list, 180,
    184–185
    as common ingredient, 73
    exchange list, 99
    Mexican-style food
    exchanges, 192
    serving sizes and
    exchanges, 100
    substitutes, 72
    vegetarian food list, 167
Rice-A-Roni dishes, 157

S

Saccharin, 43
Salad dressings, 130, 149, 153
    substitutes, 72
Salads, 157, 231–232,
234–241
Salt
    guidelines for using, 45–47
    sodium intake guidelines,
    46
    substitutes, 72
Sandwiches
    combination foods
    exchange list, 157–158
    fast food exchanges, 232,
    234–241

Saturated fats
    exchange list, 147–150
    food sources, 34–35
    ingredients with, 64
    meal planning and, 17
Sauces, 152
Sausage, 145
Scrapple, 108, 145
Seafood
    Asian food list, 182,
    184–185
    meat and meat substitutes
    exchange list, 145–146
Seeds
    fat exchange list, 149
    meat and meat substitutes
    exchange list, 146
    snack food list, 258
    vegetarian food list, 170
Serving sizes
    calculating exchanges from,
    284–285
    combination foods
    exchange list, 155
    dining out and, 78
    fat exchange list, 148
    food labeling and, 55–56
    free foods exchange list, 151
    international travel and,
    91–92
    meat and meat substitutes
    exchanges, 134–136
    in Nutrition Facts Informa-
    tion, 54–55
    other carbohydrates
    exchange list, 126
    starch exchange list, 100
Sesame Cookies, 70
Snacks
    exchange guidelines,
    249–259
    free foods exchange list,
    151–154
    meal planning with, 20–21
    other carbohydrates
    exchange list, 125–130
    starch exchange list,
    108–109, 110–111
Sodium
    dietary guidelines for,
    45–47
    ingredients with, 64
Soft drinks, 44, 130, 251–252
Soluble fibers, 48
Sorbitol, 281

Soups
    Asian food list, 180,
    184–185
    combination foods
    exchange list, 155, 158
    convenience food
    exchanges, 246
    free foods exchange list, 153
    international travel and,
    91–92
    Italian food exchanges,
    204–206
    Jewish food list, 224
    serving sizes and
    exchanges, 100
    snack food list, 258
    starch exchange list,
    109–110
    substitutes, 72
Sour cream
    fat exchange list, 150
    free foods list, 154
    substitutes, 72
Soy products
    meat and meat substitutes
    list, 146
    milk list (soy milk), 123
    vegetarian food list,
    170–171, 173
Spices, 153–154
Starches. *See also* Bread;
    Cereal; Grains; Pasta and
    noodles; Potatoes; Rice
    Asian food list, 180–181
    camping food exchanges,
    264
    common ingredients, 73–74
    exchange list, 99–111
    Indian food exchanges,
    212–218
    Italian food exchanges, 204
    Jewish food list, 222
    meal planning guidelines,
    16
    Mexican-style food
    exchanges, 192
    vegetarian food list, 167
Subway food exchanges, 240
Sucralose, 43
Sucrose, 281
Sugars
    common sugars, 279–281
    as cooking ingredient,
    75–76
    guidelines for using, 41–42
    meal planning guidelines,
    16

modifying recipes with, 67–68
reduced consumption guidelines, 44–45
sugar substitutes, 42–44
Sugar substitutes, 38, 42–44, 72
free foods exchange list, 154
Sweet acidophilus, 123
Syrups, 279–281
carbohydrating counting and, 61
as cooking ingredient, 75–76
free foods exchange list, 154
other carbohydrates exchange list, 127–130

T

Tabouli, 173
Taco Bell food exchanges, 240–241
Tahini, 149, 173
Tea, 152, 154
Tempeh
starch exchange list, 110
vegetarian food list, 171, 173
Textured vegetable protein
meat and meat substitutes list, 146
as mock duck, 187
vegetarian food list, 171, 173
Thai food exchanges and sample menus, 177, 179, 180–188
Time zones, meal planning and, 92–93
Tofu
Asian food list, 186, 188
meat and meat substitutes list, 146
vegetarian food list, 171, 173
Tortillas and tortilla chips, 111, 192, 195–197, 251–253
Trans-fatty acids, 35
Travel
information sources, 273
international travel, 90–92
meal planning and, 89–96
medical assistance during, 95–96
Tuna Helper main dishes, 159
Tuna Rice Casserole, 69

Turbinado sugar, 281
Turkey, 146
Type II diabetes, 23

V

Veal
Italian food exchanges, 206
meat and meat substitutes exchange list, 146
Vegans
defined, 163
sample menu, 166
Vegetables
Asian food list, 181–182, 186–188
calculating exchanges from, 283
camping food exchanges, 265
on starch exchange list, 106–108, 110–111
carbohydrates in, 16
as cooking ingredient, 75
as free foods, 114
Indian food exchanges, 213
Italian food exchanges, 204
Jewish food list, 223
Mexican-style food exchanges, 193
serving sizes, 113–114
substitutes, 72
vegetable exchange list, 119–120
vegetarian food list, 168
Vegetarian exchanges, 163–173
Venison, 146

W

Weight control
calories and, 19
goal setting guidelines, 28
guidelines for, 25–29
healthy weight ranges, 25–27
meal planning and, 10–11
physical activity and, 28–29
support for, 29
weight loss and, 27
Weight Watchers products, 123
Wendy's food exchanges, 241
Whipped toppings
fat exchange list, 150
free foods exchange list, 154

White Castle food exchanges, 241
Wine, 85
Worthington Foods products, 171–172

X

Xylitol, 281

Y

Yogurt
as baking/cooking ingredient, 72
carbohydrating counting and, 62
free foods list, 154
frozen yogurt, 128–129, 257
Indian food exchanges, 213–214
milk exchange list, 121–123
other carbohydrates exchange list, 128, 130
snack food list, 259
vegetarian food list, 168

Books of Related Interest from
IDC Publishing

Fast Food Facts

Fifth Edition

Marion J. Franz, MS, RD, CDE

The original book of facts on fast food, this new edition offers
readers hard-to-find nutrition information, including carbohydrate choices, food exchanges, and designated good food choices.
Recommended for anyone who frequents fast food restaurants.
Also available in a pocket edition.

Trade edition: $8.95; ISBN 1-885115-42-3
Pocket edition: $4.95; ISBN 1-885115-43-1

Convenience Food Facts

**A Quick Guide for Choosing Healthy Brand-Name Foods
in Every Aisle of the Supermarket**

Fourth Edition

Arlene Monk, RD, LD, CDE, and Nancy Cooper, RD, LD, CDE

Completely revised and expanded, *Convenience Food Facts* has
everything you need to plan quick, healthy meals using prepared
foods. This edition highlights low-fat choices among more than
3,000 popular brand-name products. Also includes carbohydrate
choices and exchange values. Ideal for anyone using a meal-
planning method to lose weight or to manage a health problem
such as diabetes.

$12.95; ISBN 1-885115-36-9

These books are available at your local bookstore.

Visit our website at www.idcpublishing.com